ISBN 978-1-949148-06-0 (Paperback Edition)

Library of Congress Control Number:

Edited by George M. Ghobrial, M.D.
Illustrated by Dakotah Justice

Printed and Bound in the USA

Published by Weatherly Press LLC
info@weatherlypress.com

AF797411

Fair Use Act Disclaimer

Osteoporosis and Compression Fractures

Diagnosis, Prevention, and Management

George M. Ghobrial, M.D.

Contents

1 Introduction

The greatest medicine of all is teaching people how not to need it. -Hippocrates

Is There an Epidemic of Osteoporosis and Fragility Fractures in North America?

Perhaps there is no medical subject that receives less attention from the media than bone density. One explanation may be that osteoporosis, a disease of low bone density, does not generate anxiety quite like cardiac disease and cancer. These two diseases are assigned by the World Health Organization (WHO) to the first and second position on the list of the most common causes of death. Nobody is born with an understanding of medicine and healthcare. Understanding the basics of modern medicine is not just for people who go to medical school. This book is the third in the *Spinal Learning Series*. Osteoporosis is one of the most neglected health care problems— it is synonymous with brittle bones. Most likely, by the end of this book, one unintentional consequence will be that osteoporosis will generate a newfound level of anxiety, as it provides a map for exploring other medical topics.

Osteoporosis does not share any special distinction as being the "most deadly". It is not a favorite of the mainstream media for that reason. It is not attention grabbing in that regard. But, as leader on "The Most Disregarded Health Conditions" list, osteoporosis is silently impacting millions of people, and it is notorious for drastically lowering quality of life.

But why is osteoporosis so disregarded? Perhaps osteoporosis is less interesting to read about because of the insidious manner of onset. How does the reader know if their bone density is declining? Dear reader, make no mistake about it, dwindling bone density is a harbinger of things to come, increasing the likelihood of fracture, chronic pain, complicated orthopedic and spinal surgeries, and a decline in overall well-being.

Most people reading this book will not seek out a book on osteoporosis for the sake of general learning. Instead, they may have a family history of osteoporosis, or have themselves been diagnosed through routine screening, or perhaps even they had a fracture and are now presented with a myriad of medications, treatments, and nebulous lifestyle advice with so many contradictions that seemingly is self-contradictory. If the reader is looking for one definitive answer on every question related to osteoporosis, this book will not provide that. This book aims to provide comprehensive and understandable education on prevention, diagnosis, management, and current and emerging therapies. However, since many healthcare experts are divided over the most ideal treatment, so will the advice be divided.

The "Ideal" Management of Bone Health is Patient-Specific

Some treatments are not appropriate for specific groups of people, due to research and data identifying elevated risk. Moreover, patients are unique, and numerous details make certain treatments more optimal for some, and suboptimal for others. Patients have allergies to certain medications— suppose a medication is identified as a forerunner in reversing osteoporosis— it is still unlikely to be given to someone with an allergy or an intolerance to that class of medication, and alternatives will be needed. Secondary osteoporosis predominantly refers to diminished bone mass and volume (osteoporosis) resulting from a particular medical problem, such as with thyroid disease, chronic medication use, or even due to strong "environmental risk factors" such as smoking and chronic alcohol abuse and malnutrition. With this in mind, it can be better understood why there is an enormous body of research, and often this information is not applicable to many people. Even for diligent researchers, years of medical training is a hurdle that will prevent nearly all people from making these decisions on their own. While this book was written in the spirit of self-education and public outreach, it is important to entrust a health care professional with support and guidance through this subject.

A Primer on Osteoporosis

Osteoporosis is a medical condition informally characterized as significantly decreased bone density and bone mass. Perhaps there is no end to how much bone loss someone can lose. However, many underlying risk factors contribute to this state of bone fragility, and in many instances, several of these risk factors may play a role in an individual's development of osteoporosis. Throughout our lives, the bone is in a constant state of balance between processes that organize and build bone, and break down bone—referred to as bone remodeling. If the balance favors breakdown, exceeding the deposition of bone, chemical and structural changes in the bone result, degrading the microstructure— over time, this leads to a fracture risk.

This is not just a frequently encountered condition in the spine clinic, it is one of the most common and insidious healthcare problems. Since fragility fractures largely impact the elderly, and the loss of bone density does not cause symptoms, most people do not prioritize preventative health advice regarding bone density. As the general age of our population steadily gets older, so has the number of "fragility fractures".

Let's suppose that the reader believes that they can proceed through life, avoiding activities that will lead to osteoporotic fractures— could it be this easy? Unfortunately, it is not. Even accidental events such as a fall from ground-level, or a motor vehicle collision can result in these fractures. To illustrate the depths to which bone density can diminish, some people do not even recall a traumatic event that caused a spine fracture. In fact, in some cases, the only even identified was some twisting movements, or they even state they woke up with back pain! Fortunately, this is less common.

Spinal Compression Fractures May Be a Harbinger of Underlying Osteoporosis

Osteoporosis is associated with fragility fractures, causing fractures anywhere in the skeleton. Among those, the most feared is a fracture of the hip (the femoral neck). Also, spinal fractures are very common as well. The most common spinal fracture related to osteoporosis is a compression fracture. Let's use a hypothetical example to illustrate a fragility fracture. In this example, a forty-year-old slipped, falling to the ground, and developed severe back pain. Ultimately, she was diagnosed with a lumbar compression fracture. This is a very common way to obtain a diagnosis of a lumbar compression fracture, but there is one feature that is less usual— her relatively young age. It is very uncommon for a person under sixty to have a spine fracture from a low-energy mechanism like this, such as a fall from the ground-level. In this instance, there is often an underlying medical condition that predisposes one to osteoporosis, either due to the condition itself (eg. thyroid disease), or the treatment (eg. chronic pulmonary disease treated with steroids). In the event of prolonged glucocorticoid exposure as a treatment of asthma, or chronic vitamin deficiency, spontaneous fractures may even occur.[1] It is also important to understand that osteoporosis is not the only cause of a spine or skeletal fracture, even in someone with obvious osteoporosis. And since some of the conditions that underly fractures can be life-threatening, such as malignancies, tumors, infection, and metabolic problems, it is important to see a physician or healthcare provider without delay to begin the process of identifying underlying etiologies.

Fragility Fractures — Bone Density in The Spine Can Deteriorate to The Point of Spontaneous Failure

Fragility fractures are caused by low energy trauma, or no trauma at all, and can occur anywhere throughout the skeleton. Insufficiency fractures are another term for a fragility fracture, and only used in the context of the sacrum, which is the rigid zone of the spine that communicates with the pelvis via large sacroiliac joints. They are also referred to as stress fractures—which can be misleading in that this has connotations of a fracture caused by an unusual level of physical activity. Sacral insufficiency fractures are often hard to identify in patients with very low bone density and can result in chronic pain when not identified. In a series of 79 patients with lumbar compression fractures requiring an invasive treatment, 10 of them were diagnosed with sacral insufficiency fractures.[2]

Bone Deterioration Can Reach Extreme Levels of Fragility, Even Younger in Life

Very few people are aware of the fullest extent to which bones can deteriorate, especially when underlying risk factors or diseases that cause osteoporosis remain undiscovered. This is evident in an extreme case of the 29 year-old woman with a four-year history of osteoporosis, who unfortunately was not able to make time for further medical workup, and in only 4 years, she sustained a sacral insufficiency fracture, just from sneezing![3] Sacral insufficiency fractures are extremely painful, and debilitating.

To be clear, this is a rare cause of a fragility fracture. Nonetheless, this extreme level of fragility is possible. Fractures in a dramatic manner like this do occur. In one study of a population of patients at-risk for osteoporosis, patients with chronic obstructive pulmonary disease (COPD), fractures were observed to occur from seemingly trivial ways such as coughing and sneezing[4], or even from a "regular" hug, causing rib fractures as well.[5] How could the bone allow itself to reach such a state? Perhaps it is because the bone is a calcium storage reservoir for the body, or a pH/ acid-base balancing system—these resevoirs can be exhausted in some conditions.

In fractures where the bone breaks with minimal effort, one way of explaining this is that the bone continues to deteriorate-until it reaches a critical point where it cannot function under minimal stress, even at rest, or without any stresses that come from minimal work, ie., walking or picking up a small box!

The Deterioration of Load-Bearing Bones

Certain bones serve load bearing functions. The cervical spine is load-bearing— it supports the skull. Likewise, the thoracic spine supports everything above it, and the lumbar spine supports an even greater load, and so on and so forth, and this load-bearing capacity increased through the lower extremities to the feet. In some instances, back pain is caused by a chronically increased load, or weight gain.

The load-bearing capacity of a bone is basically linked to the person's weight, but since there are so many causes of back pain, weight is not the only cause of back pain, and most back pain has multiple causes. Most people with back pain have an abrupt onset of back pain and are more likely to want to know what the immediate cause for worsened back pain. In chronic back pain, it can be due to more than one issue. It may be spinal or non-spinal, and it may pain due to an anatomical problem at one or more levels, or it may be a systemic medical condition presenting with back pain, such as an auto-immune condition. So, if someone's BMI is just outside of the upper limit of normal, no diagnosis has been made. The underlying causes of back pain are very complex and requires the assistance of a healthcare specialist. For the engaged reader, the author explores these questions in his book, *The Low Back Pain Guide.*

Naturally, load-bearing capacity must tolerate the increased load that comes from weight gain. Researchers have observed increased low back pain with weight loss as well, presumably from calorie reduction, ie., dieting. Other researchers have argued that there is a lack of a significant correlation between weight gain and low back pain (LBP). However, the vast majority of studies show that patients with increased weight gain are more likely to have LBP. Stone and Broderick found a higher likelihood of LBP with increasing BMI. BMI provides a context for weight and height. In their study, this relationship was consistent, regardless of age, as older patients are more likely to have back pain.[6] There is much that is not understood about LBP.

One reason why a patient with LBP uses a walker or a cane is because these assistive devices decrease the load-bearing requirements on the lumbar spine. When nerve compression is present, a walker or cane allows a patient to lean forward (flexion)— an action that could relieve nerve compression. In other instances, severe degeneration and other spinal issues, shift the center of gravity forward, and the patient becomes imbalanced. This causes chronic muscle strain and joint pain, but the cane and walker can are stabilizers that decrease muscle requirements.

Load-Bearing and Vertebral Body Failure

With respect to the skeleton, the bones of the spine are among the few bones of the body that are constantly under a load, as long as one is upright. As the amount of weight on each vertebral body increases from one level to the next, so does the size of the vertebral body. Pressure is a measure of force applied over a set area. A larger surface area would help lower the pressure on the bone. Generally, one process of arthritis, or spondylosis in the spine, is to increase the bony surface area where a load is distributed between the two joints— this keeps the pressure within a certain range. The strength of the vertebral body is dependent upon the bone mineral density, size, shape, and microstructural factors such as the distribution of different types of collagen proteins, and any ongoing microstructural injury from wear and tear, and other processes. These factors determine the overall strength of the bone, and how well it will respond to certain pressures. The bone will adapt over time to increasing pressures, and certain bones adapt better than others.

Wolff's "Law"

As discussed, the size of each vertebral body increases as one proceeds from the cervical, thoracic, and finally to the lumbar spine, which is a function of the greater amount of weight that each vertebra must carry individually, which is the cumulative mass of each vertebral body sitting above it, with additional soft tissue weight increasing this weight further. Load-bearing bone strength is thought to be guided by an internal feedback process guided by a stress response first proposed by German Surgeon and Anatomist Julius Wolff in 1892, and later expanded upon by the prolific American Orthopedic Surgeon Harold Frost with his hypothesis of the mechanostat, a proposed organic microsensor in the bone that provides feedback based on stress.[7] These are interesting ideas that distill down very complex processes in our body that are not fully understood. In essence, load-bearing bones adapt to mechanical loading, whereby the bone responds with the net result being the augmentation and reinforcement of the bone, increasing mineral density, and restructuring the microarchitecture of spongy bone that serves to increase overall strength, as well noticeable changes in the bone overall, such as thickening of the denser outer cortex of bone. Likewise, the opposite can occur when those stresses are no longer applied. If the stress decreases, the bones lose mineral density, as it were. To make matters even more complex, muscular attachments to bone apply stresses and serve as an additional route through which the bone receives feedback and an understanding of the demands of the environment.

The Environment and Bone Density- Two Extremes

The observations that mechanical stress is vital in the maintenance of bone density, as consistently observed in bed bound patients, regardless of the underlying ailment, and in other examples, observing the lack of mechanical stress with increased indirect markers of bone turnover in the blood.[8] Two intriguing examples illustrate this concept. In the first example, NASA documented their findings of the detrimental effects of chronic space exploration, being that chronic weightlessness resulted in a depletion of the bone mass. In other words, this would cause osteoporosis, and it was just a matter of how long one was in space. Note that this is a clinical scenario that statistically very few physicians will ever be able to confirm or comment on, but nonetheless, is very unique. Said NASA on their blog:

> "**In a microgravity environment, because of reduced loading stimuli**, there is increased bone resorption and no change in or possibly decreased bone formation, **leading to bone mass loss at a rate of about ten times that of osteoporosis.** The proximal femoral bone loses 1.5 percent of its mass per month, or roughly 10 percent over a six-month stay in space, with the recovery after returning to Earth taking at least three or four years. The calcium balance (the difference between intake and excretion), which is about zero on Earth, **decreases to about -250 mg**/day during flight, a value that increases the risk of kidney stones.
>
> Bisphosphonate is a therapeutic agent that has been used to treat osteoporosis patients for more than a decade, with a proven efficacy to increase bone mass and decrease the occurrence of bone fracture. Through 90-day bed rest research on Earth, we confirmed that this agent has a preventive effect on the loss of bone mass. Based on these results as well as studies conducted by others, JAXA and NASA decided to collaborate on a space biomedical

> experiment to prevent bone loss during space flight. Dr. Leblanc, USRA, and Dr. Matsumoto, Tokushima University, are the two principal investigators of this study."[9]

As seen above, the argument put forth by NASA is that the constant, "static force of gravity" is argued by NASA to be a major contributor to bone density— as its absence (by being in space) causes rapid bone mineral loss. This was also a subject discussed by NASA astronaut Scott Kelly, who wrote a book regarding his prolonged experience in space.[10]

The second fascinating example is much less exotic, but still instructive. On the opposite end of the spectrum of chronic mechanical stress correlates very high chronic stresses with very high bone density. This example is seen in elite female power lifters. The T-scores reported for a 54 year-old Caucasian woman of +2.2 and +1.9 in the lumbar spine and femoral neck, respectively, the highest ever T-score recorded in a Caucasian woman of that age.[11] These observations of very high bone density have been observed in a case series of 11 male powerlifters as well.[12] However, elevated bone mass can be observed as a measurement error, resulting from mixed density bone resulting from degenerative diseases[13] where regions of calcification and bone spurs will increase the recorded average density measurement. Also, a number of medical conditions ranging from cancer to chronic spine infections, uncommon metabolic conditions and even rare congenital conditions can lead to an elevated bone density.[14] And so, it is important to keep in mind that internal and external forces are not the most common factors affecting bone density. These examples serve to show the observations between environment, physical activity, and osteoporosis. Bone density and its responses are so complex that the greatest challenge in this book is finding clear cause-and-effect examples. For example, why do some professional athletes have decreased bone density? In some cases, it is thought there is inadequate nutrition, or hormone fluctuation resulting from chronic stresses of professional training. So then how does one determine which is the cause?

In other words, the challenge of medical research lies in finding causation amongst a sea of correlation— which in medicine is not unlike searching for the proverbial needle in a haystack. This book will discuss in detail the most important factors that impact bone density and management considerations.

The Vertebral Fracture Cascade: One Spinal Fracture Raises the Risk of Subsequent Fractures

When a vertebral body receives a load beyond the limits of its design, a compression fracture may occur. Surprisingly, after a compression fracture, there is an elevated risk for a second compression fracture in the spine. This is referred to as the "vertebral fracture cascade." The cause of this is truly a mystery that has not fully understood. It is not thought to be due to low BMD alone.[15] This phenomenon is observed more in the thoracic spine and thoracolumbar spine than anywhere else. Suffice it to say, there is some as yet unclear biomechanical change[16] that results from fracture, such as a change in how the spine distributes the load-bearing forces. Or, a deviation from normal spinal alignment could occur from a fracture, such as kyphosis, which can increase stress on certain underlying vertebra. This results in an increased risk of fracture. After the initial fracture is diagnosed, prompt action is recommended to avoid a subsequent fracture (or fractures).

Bone Fragility and Spondylosis Together May Increase Fracture Risk

As one ages, the spinal disc loses water, and degenerates. This is a process that occurs in everyone, and it is thought that the spine becomes more mobile in proportion to this degeneration. Not all disc degeneration is painful, certainly there are some that do, and quite frequently they appear undiscernible from other degenerating discs. However, some discs shorten or "collapse" with greater degrees of degeneration, and the spine responds to this increased flexibility by numerous changes that stiffens the spine— a process collectively referred to as spondylosis. These changes may include thickened ligaments, spurring, facet arthropathy, calcification of ligaments and hypertrophy of bone. As mentioned above in the preceding section, these changes may cause false measurements of increased bone density during routine screening. However, these changes do not necessarily increase overall bone strength and structural integrity as one might think. Also, these changes of spondylosis decrease spinal flexibility. To some extent, flexibility helps distribute energy, this flexibility is an operating principle in modern designs of earthquake-resistant skyscrapers as seen in these example:

> "Building on top of giant shock absorbers, ball bearings or sliding plates along with deep, flexible foundations and robust steel skeletons can help reduce the impact of powerful seismic forces and make a building earthquake-proof."[17]

Ultimately, the spine can lose flexibility and become brittle, with the bone unable to distribute the energy and breaking in a manner like chalk or a vase.

Turning back the clock to one's childhood years where falls and collisions are commonplace, the spine is able to easily distribute these very same forces, and much more, in a much more efficient and graceful manner, avoiding spinal injury and nerve damage. In a child, the flexibility of the spine and ability of the intervertebral discs to distribute shock occurs much more efficiently. As the spine becomes more and more stiff from degeneration, calcification of multiple contiguous spinal levels can lead to a fracture prone patient.

Spinal Microarchitecture is As Important as Mineralization in Avoiding Fracture

Calcium is just one essential component in the spine, and its arrangement is what truly determines strength. Most people can imagine that framing a building cannot be safely done without an understanding that there is a proper way to organize, assemble, and fasten the components. And there are better ways to do this than others, and some standards may only be suitable for different types of loads. In the spine, the microarchitecture of the bone is equally important to the density of that architecture.

Researchers have made significant progress in the past decades, but they still have much work to do before completely unraveling the mystery of the microstructure of bone and the constant process of bone turnover. Researchers aim to learn the ideal structure in hopes that to discover the true relationships between structure and fracture risk, and then ultimately what the true risk of certain lifestyle are on developing a fragility fracture.

A new grading system that identifies the ideal bone structure is a huge challenge, not just in identifying bone in a prepared bone sample, but in actually being able to develop a clinically valid grading system that is non-invasive and low risk. The current process, bone densitometry, will be discussed in detail in this book. Suffice it to say, it is considered non-invasive, however the exposure to low dose x-ray for this study is a potential risk for cancer.

Childhood and Bone Development

During childhood, it is the lack of "bone maturity" and differing makeup of proteins, and lack of spondylosis(arthritis) that makes the spine relatively more flexible than an adult. And while bone maturity and increased calcium results from a number of organizational changes and increased density, it is not only calcium that makes bones fracture-resistant. Children and adolescence have not reached their peak bone mass and are relatively resistant for reasons other than calcium. Evidence of this is seen in children who can be so fracture resistant that they can injure the nerves and/or spinal cord without evidence of damage to bones of the spine or even disc. In adults, neurologic injury without fracture or injury to the spinal disc is incredibly rare.

Hormones may be the key driver behind changes in the organization of bones. The importance of hormone exposure on bone development cannot be overstated. In fact, the tallest people in modern history, had growth hormone-secreting pituitary gland tumors, many of which grew to be over eight feet tall. Apart from length, androgens have a huge impact on bone density. Indeed, hormone deficiency is a major underlying driver of BMD loss in the case of estrogen and to a lesser extent, testosterone.

Preventative Medicine for Bone Loss

Moving on from childhood to about the third decade of life, the developing skeleton reaches its peak bone mass and skeletal maturity. From approximately the thirties and beyond, more most people, bone mass may only "go downhill" at that point—by a variety of mechanisms. Preventative medicine, the practice of avoiding disease through a healthy lifestyle— is the chief defense against bone loss. It begins with a healthy lifestyle. The reader will not be surprised to hear that smoking is a major risk factor for osteoporosis, as it impacts essential biochemical processes that underscore processes in all body functions. In isolation, there are no symptoms of the primary loss of bone density. Often, when an underlying disease process is impacting bone density, such as hyperthyroidism, a condition whereby the thyroid produces too much thyroid hormone, leads to excessive breakdown of the bone and numerous other symptoms —if left untreated will lead to osteoporosis. Even people treated with elevated doses of thyroid replacement hormone for hypothyroidism must be monitored so as not to lead to the same clinical loss of bone density. As one can see, many different medical conditions may benefit from numerous different experts as medical knowledge grows. Patients are finding themselves seeing more physicians as there are more people subspecializing, and many more healthcare providers are divesting themselves of certain diseases that are too high risk. As patients get older, often there is delay in care due to more appointments, longer wait times, and the complexities with facilitating information sharing between healthcare facilities and practices.

In many healthcare networks, decision making is getting progressively harder over time. Since there are numerous causes of secondary osteoporosis, across many subspecialities, the task of working this up can be overwhelming. Secondary osteoporosis results from an underlying disease process due to decreased bone density encompasses so many different medical problems identified that they cannot be all reasonably addressed in detail in the scope of this book. However, many will be basically illustrated.

The interested reader may consult the Center for Disease Control's (CDC) informational site on smoking titled, "Health Effects of Smoking", which gives an updated overview of the detrimental effects of smoking, with its specific impact on our different body systems, such as the lungs. Authoritative references are provided for the reader interested in understanding just exactly how these things are determined.[18] Importantly, the treatments mentioned in this book are provided as a reference for one's understanding and are not a recommendation.

References in This Book

Throughout the book, there will be numerous references provided for all of the content of this book. Wherever possible, free articles were used so that the interested reader can look up the information and learn more of the source material. When this is not the case, they will be able to look up the abstract on the National Library of Medicine's PubMed®, which is a government search engine that has access to over 33 million research articles, including some of the oldest medical literature. The National Library of Medicine also has free medical textbooks. Interesting non-scientific publications are also included as these are generally what most people are exposed to and understanding medicine often is the process of comparing publicly made claims, advertising, and news articles to published science.

Beyond this, having a full understanding of any treatment offered for any medical condition is a key component of informed consent. Informed consent is a term that encompasses many aspects of the physician-patient relationship and the process of receiving any type of medical care. For a brief overview of informed consent, one can read about the history of informed consent, and the fundamental components as well as commonly encountered barriers, such as education. These resources are freely accessed online and provided through both government[19,20] and private resources.[21,22]

Should they determine they have a disorder of decreased bone density such as osteopenia or osteoporosis, they will then undergo medical treatment. This involves treatment with medications and lifestyle modification to avoid the identified behaviors that contribute to the loss of bone density. However, these life styles lead to the slow loss in bone density in years for more people, in tandem with genetic predispositions of those with a fair-complexion of European descent.

Last, for those patients who unfortunately were unable to prevent a fracture from occurring, there are medical treatments, interventional treatments such as vertebroplasty and kyphoplasty to discuss, and then briefly, in the severest instances, there are spinal surgical treatments for osteoporotic fractures of the spine. These will be briefly discussed for a general understanding. If the reader fell in the latter category they would have already undergone treatment by the time they decided to find books and educate themselves on the subject.

Overall, healthcare is an increasingly complex world, , that cannot be navigated without the help of family and friends who can be of assistance in discussing treatment options, lifestyle goals, and lending emotional support along the journey. Perhaps equally important is the need to find in advance a physician or other healthcare provider who the reader trusts that will help them in making the decision that takes into consideration one's goals and values, and helps them make the most informed decision.

How to Use This Book

Before expanding upon the very exciting topics related to osteoporosis, the author understands that reading cover-to-cover may not be ideal for a healthcare book. Previously, in *The Low Back Pain Guide* and *The Neck Pain Guide*, these books were organized more in the question-and-answer reference format. In this, the book is organized by major knowledge areas of osteoporosis, such as prevention, diagnosis, and treatments. It is recommended to consult the table of contents as all of the subheadings are included which includes many specific topics within each subheading. If there is even more detail one is searching for, a comprehensive index is located at the end.

For patients that have an interest in preventative health, the author highly recommends a careful read of the book from cover-to-cover. However, perhaps the reader only has specific questions, such as inquiring about a recommendation for a bone density screening, which will be discussed in the diagnostics section of this book. In any case, if time is limited, refer to the necessary sections and live a healthier life!

2 A Brief Overview of the Spine

The spine consists of multiple vertebrae, connected by intervertebral discs, which together form a support column that extends from the skull to the pelvis. Each individual vertebra is a cylindrical block of bone containing a right and left extension of bone called pedicles, that articulate to facet joints (figure).

The Spine

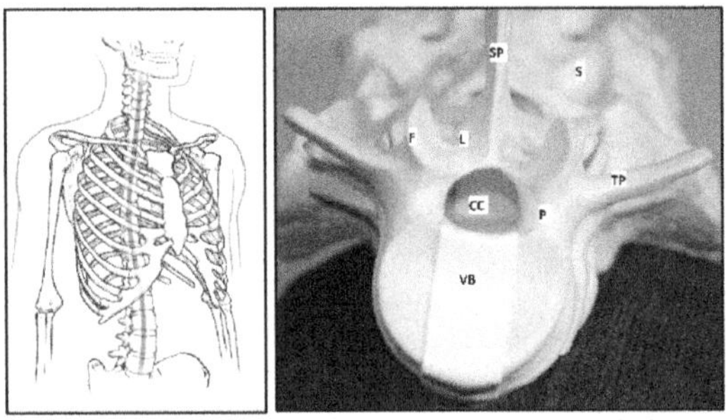

Figure 1 The Mobile Spine (left image) consists of the cervical, thoracic and lumbar segments. Each individdual segment consists of a cylindrical support segment of bone, called a vertebral body (VB, right image of the lumbar spine, superior view). With the right and left pedicles (P), and the paired facets (F), lamina (L), and spinous process (SP), a concentric ring is formed around a central canal (CC). The central canal transmits the nerves and spinal cord (not shown). Part of the sacrum (S) can be seen below the lumbar spine, which provides a connects from the spine to the pelvis. Left image reprinted from The Low Back Pain Handbook (2019, Ghobrial).

All of these structures form a hollow ring whereby this central channel allows for the protection of the spinal cord and nerve roots. The fact that the spinal cord and nerves are protected by bone serves as evidence of their degree of importance, and also there fragility. Spinal nerves exit the spinal cord and exit via foramina, which is an opening created on the left and right sides, between two vertebral bodies, with the exception of the unique bones adjacent to the skull. In the author's previous books, *The Low Back Pain Book (2019), and The Neck Pain Book (2020)*, back and extremity pain caused by nerve compression is explained in detail. Suffice it to say, time, or aging of the spine, is the predominant cause of degeneration[1] that ultimately causes the narrowing of these bony foramina in the spinal canal, leading to pain and even weakness and numbness due to nerve and spinal cord compression.

Global Spinal Alignment and Pain

The local relationship between one nerve and the adjacent vertebral body, pedicles, facets, and disc is of course important, but the relationship between the overall spinal curvature is equally important. Without balance, pain and disability will result. The spine is balanced in such a way that allows for us to stand upright, expending as little energy as possible in maintaining our balance. In other words, it should not be a struggle to stand upright, neither should it be painful, or lead to imbalance on our feet, or be a cause for chronic pain.

Our body maintains this upright posture and balance as one can visualize a scale. This scale is slightly different in that one side of the scale is a weight, and the other side is like a series of suspension cables on a bridge. The one side of the scale, in front

---

[1] There are numerous terms that either describe the same exact process of spondylosis, or a subset of processes that contribute to spondylosis. Degenerative spinal disorders is a catch-all phrase that includes the above, disc herniations, and many other phrases. This overlap can contribute to confusion with patients as health care professionals may describe the same condition using a number of terms.

of the spine (anterior), are our organs, ribs, chest, and abdomen, along with its contents (organs, blood vessels, and other soft tissues). Almost all of the body's muscle mass is situated behind (posterior) the spine, where there are thousands of small and large muscular attachments that pull on the spine. Standing straight involves a contraction of these muscles, which pulls on these bones (also called the posterior elements), extending the body. When a person bends forward, the spine flexes, which is the opposite of extension.

Imbalance of the spine can occur in either of three ways. For many people, this upset balance occurs by an increase in overall body weight, where fat deposition occurs in the abdominal region which leads to a shifting of the center of gravity in front of the feet, upsetting the balance. In some people, the loss of posterior musculature can occur, also upsetting this balance.

Perhaps more commonly than that, and most relevant to this book, is the change in the structure of the spine causing this forward shift in center of gravity. As will be discussed below, the disc will degenerate over time, shortening the front of the spine, causing it to pitch forward. This happens to all people. This will also occur with compression fractures, where the bone is shortening as well. The net result is to take the balance spine and to tip it forward, which requires a lot of effort to balance. One can also imagine the problems that are created by walking.

When a person has nerve compression, perhaps from a disc herniation, the natural response is to lean forwards, as it alleviates nerve compression. Separating spinal stenosis and resulting nerve compression from a person with a spinal imbalance as we discussed above is very important because the treatments are two entirely different approaches. This is one more issue underscoring the complexities of diagnosing and treating spinal diseases.

Last, if one is wondering why the author did not discuss the other state, the shift in center of gravity to behind the spine (posterior), the negative sagittal balance, fortunately, this is rare and an esoteric subject. If the problem were severe enough, this would create a propensity to fall backwards, if this exceeded one's ability to lean forwards, which can happen in some instances. This would be something the reader would never forget if they saw it. Again, this is a rare occurrence, but for the highly curious reader, this issue has been examined in the medical literature.[23]

Spinal Anatomy

Oriented from "highest to lowest", the cervical is located in the neck, the thoracic in the torso, and lumbar spine in the abdomen — which are the flexible, or mobile regions of the spine. The presence of joints between these levels are what constitutes to that flexibility. The difference in mobility is attributed to the unique anatomy of each joint and region of the body described above, and is a complex matter— overall, out of the scope of this book. The unique anatomical features will be discussed as necessary for the relevance of osteoporosis.

The cervical spine consists of seven vertebral segments, while the thoracic consists of twelve, and the lumbar spine consists of five. Below the flexible spine are the fixed sacral and coccygeal regions. These regions have no flexibility because they lack discs. The entire sacral segment is a region of five segments that are fused together during development. Each sacral segments however, as with all other segments of the spine, contains an opening on the right and left side for a pair of nerve roots to exit, one on each side. This opening is referred to as a neural foramen (pl. foramina). In the coccygeal segment, there are usually 4 segments. Overall, it is widely reported that there are 33 spinal segments, as this represents most people.

The Spine

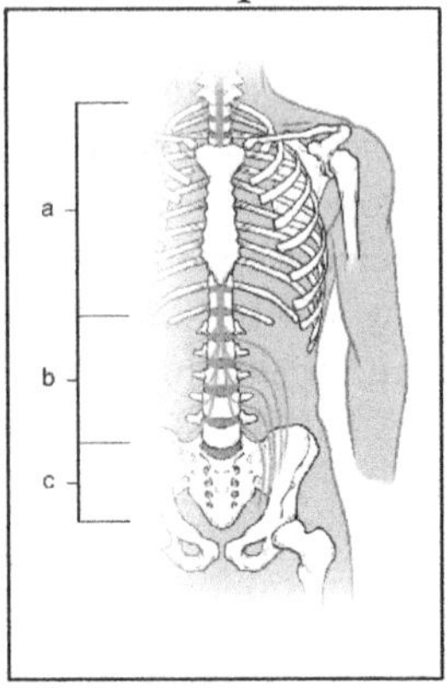

Figure 2: The Spine. (left) The spine is anatomically divided by structure and function: (a) thoracic, (b) lumbar, (c) sacrum. The cervical spine is found above the thoracic spine and is located in the neck, connecting the base of the skull to the first thoracic vertebra. (right) Oblique view of the spine showing its central position in the skeleton for weight-bearing, locomotion, and transmitting the nerves to and from the spinal cord, protected by the spine (Figure Source: The Low Back Pain Book, Ghobrial, 2019).

Individual Variations in The Anatomy of The Spine

It may surprise the reader that consistency in spinal anatomy is not always maintained, from one person, to the next. Typically, inconsistencies in the interrelationships of body structures are summarily viewed as abnormal and thought to be due to genetics, viz., that these are abnormal genetics.[24] But since modern science has a long way to go in terms of deciphering the true purpose of the genetic code, for the present, nonprotein coding DNA, ie. the DNA of unknown purpose, is contemptuously called "junk" DNA. And over time, as the role of DNA is understood, as well as other forms of genetic information, the amount of "junk" is reclassified. As it stands, less than 2% of the genetic code is understood.

In likewise fashion, variations in anatomy receive labels such as supernumerary, vestigial, a disorder, or malformation. As with DNA, a lack of knowledge of the existence of a function of an anatomical structure leads to dismissal of any importance.

And in the case of these structures, they are labeled "vestigial". Exactly how much longer this label will persist is unknown, due to the growing countercurrent of dissenting scientist resulting from the steady advancement in medical knowledge.[25]

For some anatomical details, variations are present in over 20-30% of people, and many of these variations are not abnormal, and most of these are not disease causing. In these instances, what makes anatomy regular, other than by majority consensus? In the modern diagnosis of bone mineral density, a chief diagnostic tool is the bone densitometry which relies on a scale that set the average density at zero— more on this in the subsequent diagnostic section. Is "above average" okay for all individuals, or do they need more? This will be explored later. In matters where the clinical significance of this variation is unknown, this is problematic. The spine contains a number of interesting variants, many of which the significance is unknown, although loosely observed in some instances with certain degenerative conditions of the spine. However, by no means does this suggest that the spine contains any structures comparable to wisdom teeth and tonsils, which are excised. This truly is a complicated topic, but several examples should help clarify the issue further.

The Coccyx

The inferior-most (lowest) spine, the coccyx, which is known to most as the "tailbone" is not a vestigial tail, but serves its function in sitting, and providing a site of muscular attachment essential to both sitting and the pelvic floor. One treatment of last resort for intractable tailbone-region pain, the coccygectomy, is reserved for persistent pain, often due to chronic pain after a fracture. The removal of this bone in many patients results in satisfactory pain relief. However, this is not meant to serve as evidence that the "tailbone" may be removed without functional consequence. And, the tailbone region is unlikely to be a remnant of an actual tail, although some scientists have made this claim in the absence of proof, other than observing It may interest the reader that there are dozens of cases reported in the literature on what is termed a "true tail" and even a "pseudo-tail"— interesting, but both are rare developmental abnormalities.[26] Nonetheless, the coccyx is referred to as the tailbone, but serves an important function.

The coccyx ostensibly has several "variants"— not to be confused with the use of variants in describing infectious diseases. In one imaging study, CT scans obtained of the coccyx as part of routine imaging for non-spinal problems, showed different numbers of coccygeal segments: 3 coccygeal segments in 13%, 4 in 76%, and 5 in 11% of participants.[27] As with most anatomy, normally anatomy is assigned the role to the most common of the variations, which is that the coccyx is agreed to have 4 segments. Not only that, there are various anatomical configurations/shapes that coccyx may take, some thought to be more associated with pain than others. As one can see, identifying the cause of pain, were that pain to be 100% associated with a single cause, is very complex. Usually, pain, especially chronic pain, has more than one origin.

Lumbar

The "low back" is most commonly associated with the lumbar spine. The lumbar spine is mobile, and it's fifth and lowest segment articulates with the first sacral vertebral body. The sacrum is non-mobile and serves as a transition point for distributed weight from the spine to the pelvis. Anatomical variations are also found in the lowest mobile disc space, which is the disc between the fifth lumbar and first sacral segment. This transitional anatomy is clinically important to patients important to physicians.

Transitional lumbar anatomy has several variants, depending on the classification systems used. Since a larger number of people have this variant anatomy, naming spinal levels, if not consistent, can generate confusion when there is a lack of agreement between radiologists who create written imaging reports using inconsistent labelling. For example, one report may refer to L5, while the other uses the label L4 for the same exact level. One can imagine the level of confusion this can generate. Select reports estimate that 3.9 to 35% of the population has variant lumbosacral anatomy.[28-30] Studies of the coccyx and lumbosacral junction region are relevant because of their association with pain. This is different than saying this is a cause of pain, but just an observation. In one study of young men, low back pain was more commonly associated with transitional lumbosacral anatomy.[31] Examples of this include an extra lumbar vertebra (six lumbar vertebra instead of five), a 13th rib (lumbar rib, instead of 12 ribs), a "lumbarized" sacrum where the first sacral segment fails to fuse to the sacrum, and a "sacralized" lumbar segment where the fifth lumbar vertebra fuses to the sacrum. As mentioned before, not only are these issues complex and associated with pain, but they present a challenge for clinical care due to the use of different labels by different practitioners.

Due to the number of variants, its complexity, and interesting anatomy, this is the extent of detail that will be discussed in this book for the present purposes. Rather, for the present, the key anatomical characteristics of the lumbar spine to understand is the relationship between exiting nerve roots and how they travel in proximity to the bony bridges called pedicles, and the intervertebral disc, as well as some basic structure and function (See Figures below).

Lumbosacral Spinal Anatomy, Posterior and Anterior Views

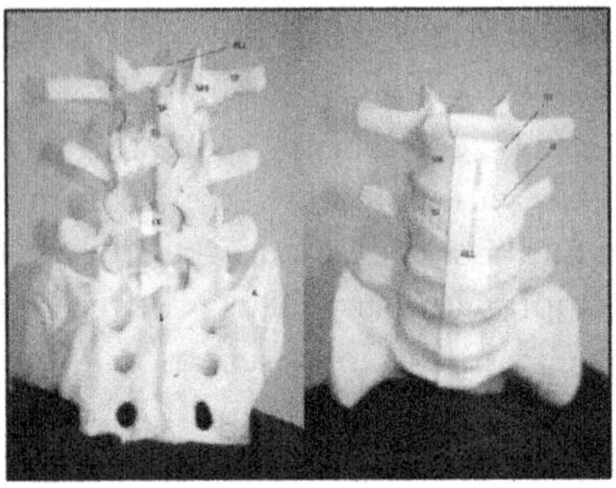

Figure 3. Posterior (left) and anterior (right) view of the lumbosacral spinal anatomy using a Sawbones Model. PLL, posterior longitudinal ligament; TP, transverse process; MB, mamillary bodies; SP, spinous process; L, lamina; CC, central canal; S, sacrum; SE, superior endplate of the vertebral body (VB); IE, inferior endplate; ID, intervertebral disc; ALL, anterior longitudinal ligament.

A posterior view of the spine basically refers to a view from behind, while an anterior view is the opposite, lateral is exactly 90 degrees off from that ("a side view"), and oblique is anywhere in between anterior and lateral. In the posterior view of this spine model, one can visualize the respective layers as one travels deeper towards the spine: the skin, fatty soft tissue, a tough fascial layer, and the many paraspinal muscles. Within the spine model, there are no ligaments or nerves shown. As seen from the anterior view, one can imagine the abdominal contents in between the skin and the anterior aspect of the spine. "In-front" of the spine, or, anterior to the transverse processes (labelled "TP" in the figures above) is where the abdomen is located, along with the aorta and large psoas muscles that aid in stability and for walking (not shown).

In the next image, a superior view is seen, which is a view looking down, the central canal can be seen (see figure below). In the cervical and thoracic spine, a spinal cord would be seen in the central canal, surrounded by a fluid-filled sac, enclosed by a membrane called that dura, filled with cerebrospinal fluid created in the brain. The spinal cord terminates at the level of the first lumbar vertebral body in most people, and paired nerves exit at each level.

Lumbosacral Spine Anatomy, Superior view

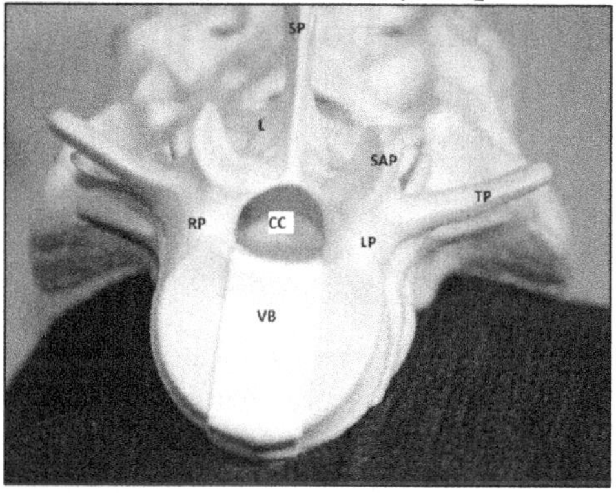

Figure 4. Lumbosacral Spinal Anatomy, Superior, or Bird's Eye View of the bony anatomy. L, lamina; SAP, superior articular process of the facet; TP, transverse process; RP, right pedicle; LP, left pedicle; VB, vertebral body; CC, central canal; SP spinous process.

Lumbar Spinal Anatomy, Lateral View

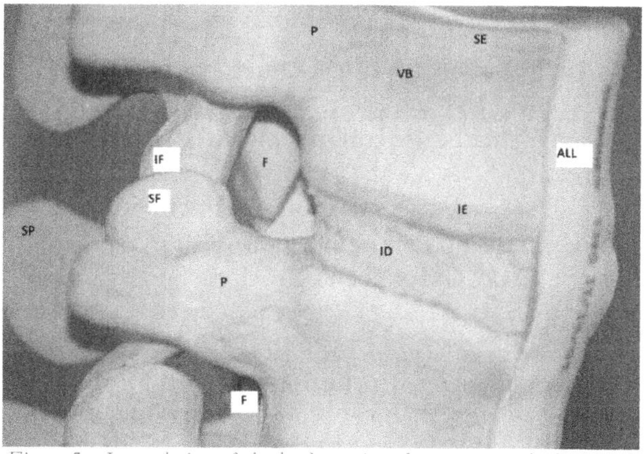

Figure 5. Lateral view of the lumbar spine, demonstrating the bony anatomical relationships in relation to the neural foramen. P, pedicle; SE, superior endplate; IE, inferior endplate; VB, vertebral body; ALL, anterior longitudinal ligament; F, neural foramen; SP, spinous process; ID, intervertebral disc, SF, superior facet, IF, inferior facet

3 Osteoporosis Bone Quality and Health

Bone quality is a subjective term because it lacks a specific measurement scale. There is no definition for "good" or "satisfactory" bone quality. We all have in our minds an idea of what this means. If someone was asked to envision what "quality" bone was: perhaps most people would provide a similar explanation: lasts a long time, and obviously bone that maintains its structure throughout one's lifetime, without fail (ie. spine fracture). The relatively "higher" the quality, the more resistant to fracture one would be. With excellent bone quality, one would envision that there would be "zero risk" of spontaneous fracture.

In the present age, for scientists, the concept of bone quality is becoming less and less of a mystery. Generally, bone quality is thought to be determined by the bony architecture at the microscopic level, the rate and quality of turnover or remodeling, any accumulation of structure injury, the mineral content, and also the composition, quantity, and arrangement of the proteins and minerals such as collagen and calcium, respectively.[32]

Bone provides structure and support for the whole body—it is the skeleton. Lumber is used to build a homes, and provides structure and support (note the different spelling of lumber). The degradation of either lumber in your home, or your lumbar vertebra can have devastating consequences for your health. That is about where the similarities end in the context of osteoporosis. Remodeling of bone occurs daily, throughout life, and is a living structure, not just deposits of calcium and other minerals.

On the surface, this process of "building up" and "breaking down" is seemingly antagonistic as a consequence of their diametrically opposed action— wasteful as well. Except, this is not the case. Basically, as with muscle, bone may be broken down over time. Micro-injury to daily stress is similar in both muscle and bone, and the body has a process for rebuilding these tissues to maintain, or to augment out of a necessity to meet greater demands. The first process in bone turnover is bone deposition, which occurs via the action of cells called osteoblasts. The antagonizing force breaks down bone, through the action of cells called osteoclasts. This common model is becoming increasingly more complex over time, as there are regulatory and intermediary processes identified all the time. And for those that want to read about the "other cells" involved, several concise reviews are available online where the purposes of the osteocytes and bone lining cells are described, and how the bone acts in the manner of a large organ system—interacting with other organs through signaling, regulating the level of acidity in our blood, calcium, and more.[33]

Interestingly, more recently, this process of remodeling has been characterized as occurring within a specialized vascular compartment called the bone remodeling compartment (BRC).[34] The vertebral bodies are closely connected to our blood supply, serving as a lesser location for hematopoiesis, ie., production of components of our blood. Also, the rich blood supply of this bone serves as a route by which hormones may stimulate bone growth.

Within this compartment, regulatory factors such as key hormones involved with bone development such as parathyroid hormone, growth hormone, testosterone and estrogen can impact the state of bone turnover. For example, one disorder of excess bone growth is due to excessive growth hormone exposure during adolescence, prior to the closure of the growth plates in our long bones. Gigantism is a condition due to growth hormone exposure and is responsible for the "giants of our modern times", accounting for the modern record. Let's briefly examine the example of the tallest man in recorded history, who reached eight feet, eleven inches (see figure below).

The '8 11" Tall Alton Giant: Growth Hormone and The Capacity for Bone Growth

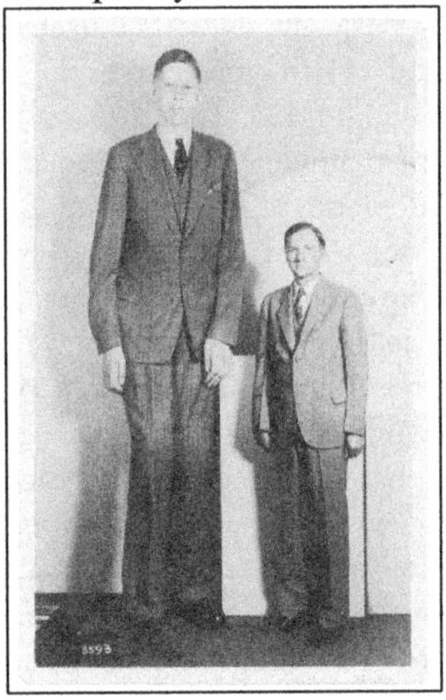

Figure 6. Robert Wadlow (1918-1940)[35] is considered to be the tallest person in recorded history, who grew to the height of 8 foot, 11 inches tall, and is photographed with his father. Due to oversecretion of growth hormone, a shortened life is tragically, very common for people with gigantism, most often due to cardiopulmonary failure. He passed away at age 22, and it was thought that due to high levels of growth hormone he was still getting taller at age 22. He was taller than his father (seen on right) at age 8, and at age 21, he was 491 pounds, and as the photo shows, this is all lean body mass. The growth hormone exposure made him powerful, and he could effortlessly lift a few hundred pounds.

This example was meant to illustrate the power of the hormone feedback mechanism, and how a growth hormone tumor did not respond to the normal negative feedback that would shut off growth hormone production. Much of childhood and adolescence is guided by hormone levels. Once an individual reached the twenties in their life, they reach a peak bone mass. In general, the following the table lists in brief, the classes of hormones that impact bone development. The treatment of bone density with hormonal replacement therapy is very complex and should be done under the direction of a trained physician. Often, in the case of complex medical issues, management of these issues is guided by an endocrinologist, a physician specializing in disorders of the endocrine system (ie. problems of hormone regulation).

Hormones Regulating Bone Density

Hormone	**Net Effect on BMD* (+/-)**
Estrogen	(+) Decreases bone loss: protects bone from resorption of parathyroid hormone, increases bone deposition activity (of osteoblasts), and decreases bone breakdown (by osteoclasts).
Parathyroid Hormone	(-) Increases bone breakdown (net effect is to increase osteoclast activity)
Calcitonin	(+) Decreases bone breakdown (by inhibiting osteoclasts)
Thyroxine	(-) Increases bone breakdown by stimulating osteoclasts.
Testosterone	(+) Decreased bone breakdown (in men)[36]
Growth Hormone	(+) Increases bone deposition[37]

**Bone mineral density*

Osteoporosis and Spinal Compromise

The spine is a critical weight-bearing structure, and the loss of bone density can cause spontaneous structural failure. Even a spontaneous pancake collapse of one segment is possible—without trauma, ie., without even falling to the ground! Fortunately, a spontaneous collapse is relatively less common, requiring very severe osteoporosis.

The Vertebra

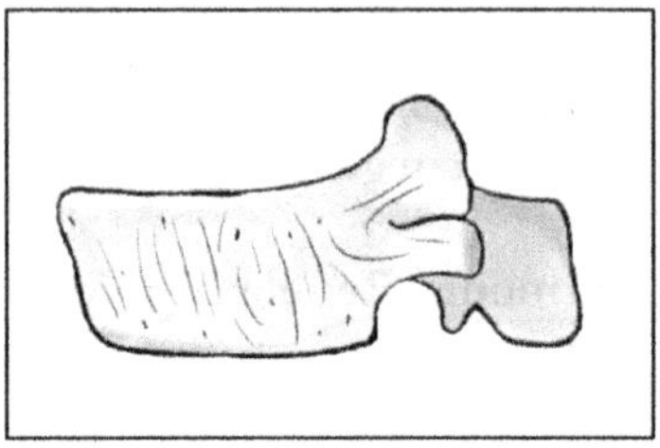

Figure 7 The Vertebra. The main load bearing unit of the spine is the vertebral body (VB). There are 5 lumbar, 12 thoracic, and 7 cervical vertebral bodies in most people.

Interestingly, despite the fact that humans are bipedal, meaning that they walk upright, the biomechanics of the vertebral body does not differ substantially from many quadrupedal animals. Several biomechanical studies have been performed using different animal models. This includes sheep, pig, goat, calf, baboon, deer, and dog.[38] However, nuances have been observed, and despite these differences between animals and humans, such as the larger average vertebral body height seen with goats and sheep relative to humans, animal models are generally considered to be useful biomechanical analogues to humans.[39] In other words, they are similar enough to be considered useful for scientific research and the studies provide useful insights into human biomechanics.

The Vertebral Body – Soup Can Analogy

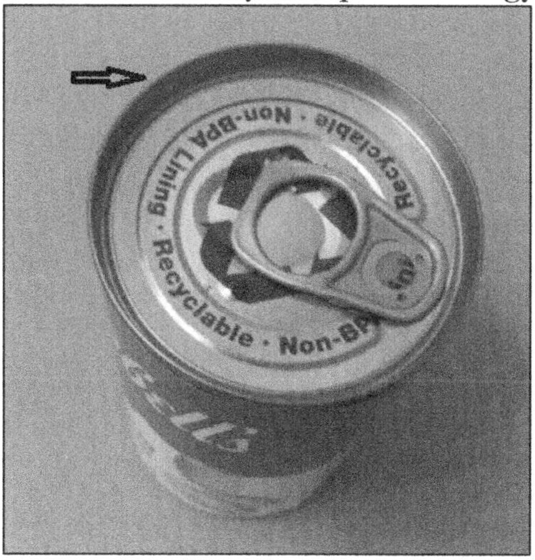

Figure 8: Spinal Structure and Load-Bearing. The rim of a metal soup can (arrow) is analogous to the bony ring of the vertebral endplate called the apophyseal ring, whereby in both the can and the vertebra, there is greater is greater cortical bone density and resistance to compression failure amongst the periphery.

Load-Bearing Forces, Illustrated

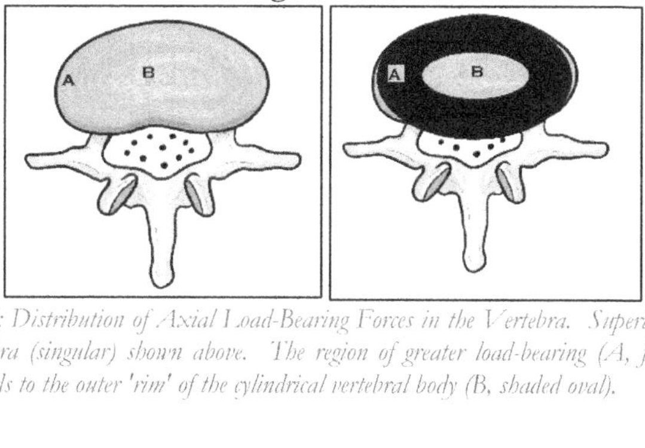

Figure 9: Distribution of Axial Load-Bearing Forces in the Vertebra. Superior view of the vertebra (singular) shown above. The region of greater load-bearing (A, figure left) corresponds to the outer 'rim' of the cylindrical vertebral body (B, shaded oval).

As seen in the aforementioned figures, the resistance of the vertebral body to compression forces is relatively greatest towards the periphery where the apophyseal ring is located. The strength is relatively less in the center of the endplate and trabecular bone. Also, trabecular bone accounts for only 20% of the bone mass of the vertebral body, and is relatively less dense than the outer cortical bone.[40] Regarding the differences between trabecular and cortical bone, Mittra writes:

> "Besides apparent density, stiffness and strength of cortical and trabecular bone depend on the loading direction, indicating its anisotropic microstructure. In general, bone can resist to higher compression loads than tension loads and to higher tension loads than shear loads. In line with this, the **trabecular connectivity inside a bone – as a measure of anisotropy – contributes more to the bone's biomechanical strength than the trabecular thickness or the bone mineral density.**"[41] (emphasis added)

Indeed, it is not only calcium content and mineralization that determines biomechanics. Also, the lack of uniformity of the trabecular bone in a single vertebra results in a variation of the BMD of a factor of up to 100.[41]

Osteoporosis – Changes in the Vertebral Body

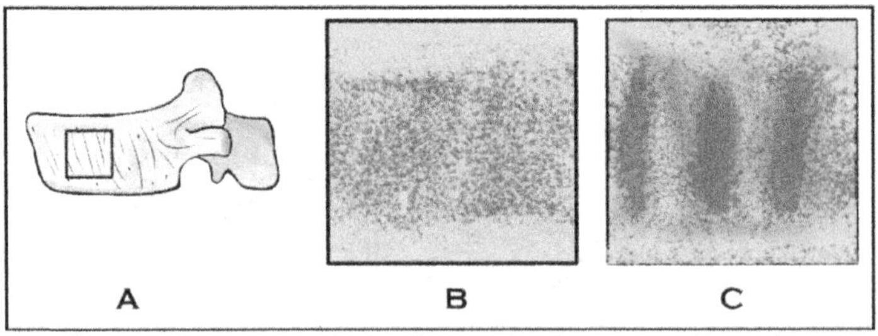

Figure 10 Osteoporosis is the degradation of the microstructure of bone. A: vertebral body illustration, trabecular bone, no magnification. B. Magnified view showing relatively normal marrow, and depletion of the vertebral marrow (C).

4 Osteoporosis, The Public Health Crisis

Osteoporosis is incredibly common; This disease of bone deterioration results in 2 million fractures annually. The economic costs for osteoporosis is rising as well, although purchasing parity, inflation, and standards of healthcare practice are never constant. All of this presents as a challenge to comparing the results of economic studies. A few studies will be presented for consideration. The annual cost of caring for osteoporosis in the US was estimated to be 17 billion USD in 2005.[42] And yet, in another study, there was an estimated annual expense of 10-15 billion US dollars in 2016.[43] In another study, this expense was projected to reach $25.3 billion by 2025.[44] These financial studies will always vary, and it leaves both the uninitiated and the healthcare professional alike, scratching their heads, wondering how calculations can be billions off. The key point is that this is a huge financial expense. Also, these numbers are always going to be conservative due to the challenges of capturing all patients in a study. Also, these studies will always fail to account for the true costs, as they are limited to the direct financial costs, such as the costs of healthcare charges.

Considering indirect costs would include lost productive years in the work force from disability, and a whole trove of additional unforeseen expenses such as legal and financial ramifications. Applying other definitions of indirect costs (or even indirect costing), and one gets a sense that the true cost is far higher.

The Prevalence of Osteoporosis

Overall, it is estimated that over 700,000 Americans each year are negatively impacted by osteoporosis, resulting in 66,000 office visits and close to 70,000 hospitalizations each year.[43] In a related United States Preventative Task Force (USPTF) survey, over 12 million individuals over the age of 50 were affected by osteoporosis.[45] Of these millions of osteoporotic fractures, 71% occur in women. At any age, osteoporotic fractures are more likely to occur in women.[44] In other estimates by the National Osteoporosis Foundation, when individuals with low bone mass, or osteopenia are included, these figures skyrocket to 54 million people in the US, which is one out of every 8 persons, or approximately 12.5% of the 2021 population.

The Silent Nature of Osteoporosis

The dangers of osteoporosis lie in its silent course. And as a result, many people will heed the warnings of the dangers of osteoporosis. They will not consider a "clinically silent" disease like this of high importance— one which does not cause any noticeable symptoms throughout life. As a reminder, the calamity of these clinically silent diseases lies in the progression of irreversible tissue damage. One fateful day, debilitating manifestations occur, and finally bringing concern with it. But by this time it is sadly too late, as the havoc of uncontrolled hypertension and diabetes has caused irreversible destruction via atherosclerosis.

Due to the lack of public interest in healthcare prevention processes during our "prime years", it is hard to know the true percentage of our population that is affected. The author's best guess is that it is higher than what is measured. In a report of the surgeon general, it is estimated that 4 out of every 10 Caucasian women over the age of 50 will have a hip, spine, or vertebral column fracture at some point in life.[46] **In one study of 758 patients over age 60 with hip fractures, the mortality**

recorded during the first 12 months was approximately 21%, or 161 people.[47] In other words, approximately 1 out of every five was dead by the end of the 12 month observation period.

Retrospective and Prospective Studies, a Brief Overview

A brief digression is required regarding two study designs, which is important as many studies reference the study design in the study title. The aforementioned hip fracture study was a retrospective one, meaning the data had already been collected and organized by the time the study was proposed. Often data can be collected (with patient and institution permission always) for the purposes of more than one future study. This type of design, a *retrospectively designed* study, is considered a major flaw among research studies. In *prospectively designed* studies, data collection follows the design of the study. This is considered more optimal as more relevant data can be collected. Also, the percentage of complications and even death is often reported to be higher, demonstrating how superior study design can provide more comprehensive data. The most likely reason is that this type of study is designed in advance— specifically so as not to overlook details. Studies have found that retrospectively collected data are associated with reporting a lower complication rate, as compared with those that are prospectively collected.[48]

Unsurprisingly, retrospective studies often suffers from limited follow-up information. Contacting patients on the database for follow-up is usually incomplete, and any additional measured outcomes not in the original database are not available for every patient. For example, even determining if patients on a ten-year old database are available for a follow-up questionnaire, or even if they are deceased, can often be a difficult to determine. The accuracy of data collected outside of a researcher's knowledge adds additional uncertainty.

As such, differences in study design largely account for the huge range in mortality reported for patients with a hip fracture, which was reported to be 14 to 58% in the first year![49] Most people will be surprised to find out that osteoporotic fractures are a major cause of disability and some fractures even can cause early death, as well as result in major depression, decreased activity, loss of independence (nursing care needed), and other medical complications associated with inactivity such as skin breakdown (pressure ulcers) and blood clots (thrombosis).

5 Preventative Health

While there are many features of osteoporosis that are not understood with a high degree of certainty, one's lifestyle is thought to play an important role in modifying their risk for the development of osteoporosis. Lifestyle factors commonly include morbid obesity (BMI > 40), chronic alcohol use, and smoking. A change in lifestyle if made early enough, can make a huge impact on improving peak adult bone mass and also maintaining it.

Clinical Research Findings and Osteoporosis

In general, several large, well-funded studies have provided useful information about the impact of lifestyle on disease. These studies are prospectively-designed. Later on, due to the high data collection standards of these studies, new questions were asked and applied to the old databases. Whether or not this truly is classified as retrospective is an interesting topic for the inquisitive reader. High-quality prospective studies are incredibly expensive and a financial barrier to conducting research. For now, it's important to understand that there is a distinction, which can potentially limit the quality of the data.

With that in mind, on the most frequently utilized databases is the Framingham Heart Study. For our purposes, the Framingham Osteoporosis Study is a study looking at risk factors for osteoporosis, utilizing data from the Framingham Heart Study.[48] This study was conducted over 4 years, measuring bone mineral density (BMD) between 1988-89 and 1992-93. A variety of potential risk factors were assessed using bone densitometry and a number of non-standard imaging technologies to assess bone quality. Ultimately, additional data was collected and this was not merely the repurposing of a former study. In addition, blood work was (serum markers) were collected, nutrition, and diet were further collected by survey questionnaire to assess diet and its relationship with BMD.[50]

The authors found an average BMD decline that was greater in women (3.4-4.8%) than in men (0.2-3.6%), irrespective of the specific bone in the skeleton that was analyzed across the 4-year interim. The standard bones analyzed include the left femoral neck ("hip"), lumbar spine, and the wrist. BMD declined regardless of gender. Several associations with BMD loss were identified in women. These were underweight people, interim weight loss, and increased alcohol consumption. Interestingly, those with interim 4-year weight gain tended to have a gain in BMD or little if any changes in BMD. The use of estrogen appears to be protective for women —resulting in less of a decline in BMD, whereas women who did not use estrogen saw a relatively greater decline in BMD by 2.7%. Weight loss appeared to also be a risk factor for men, and also weight gain appeared to be protective. Other risk factors identified in men included smoking, inactivity, low vitamin D (specifically serum 25-OH vitamin D), and low calcium intake.

These are quite a few findings, but they are also incomplete. Without a more complete assessment, these aforementioned lifestyles are vague generalizations. The specifics are missing, such as how much exercise, what kind, and for how long, need to be addressed. The importance of diet, tobacco use, vitamin intake, and exercise will now all be examined in detail. Doing so would be akin to taking the reader into the wilderness and dropping them off, without any map or guidance whatsoever. Almost every week, one hears about new health risks, or how our understanding of risk has changed.

Smoking, Nicotine, and Bone Health

With over forty million tobacco smokers, tobacco consumption is the leading preventable cause of disease, disability, and death in the United States.[51] For the very efficient thinker, perhaps the easiest way to understand tobacco and bone loss is that you necessarily have to, since it is the leading cause of preventable disease, disability, and death. Tobacco use has never been shown to increase bone density.

Nonetheless, it is not well known that both nicotine as well as tobacco smoking both contribute to the development of osteoporosis. For many people, quitting smoking involves the transition from smoking to another nicotine product. This is a major achievement. This is something that is very difficult to do, and often it is a battle of multiple relapses. As mentioned, there are numerous health benefits for those who hang in there through each and every battle.

Unfortunately, for those switching to nicotine, there is still more progress to be made. Available laboratory evidence suggests that nicotine lowers BMD. Numerous independent rat studies have shown that nicotine is associated with bone density loss, when compared with the control rat population that had no nicotine exposure.[52,53] Researchers have even uncovered a mechanism for how nicotine lowers BMD. Recent work suggests that a specific receptor in the bone may be bound by nicotine, negatively influencing bone turnover.[54]

Smoking exposes the cells of the bones to much more than nicotine. Nicotine, chemical additives, and free radicals are implicated in the impact on bone turnover. The result is a bone remodeling process that favors bone breakdown. Perhaps a remodeling occurs that decreases structural integrity, not just bone density. This is a prevailing opinion, despite there being knowledge gaps regarding the underlying biomolecular mechanisms.[55]

Cellular processes are dynamic. In other words, numerous positive- and negative- feedback mechanisms regulate the activation, deactivation, and rate of these processes. Is there a way by which all of these processes may be simultaneously monitored in the living cell by a researcher? Unfortunately, these techniques are only recently developed and only offer a narrow glimpse. It is only a matter of time.

Without too much of a digression, to give the reader a sense of how much modern science knows about the cell, one can read about the history of "junk DNA", which was the term given to DNA without any known function. The percentage of junk contained in our genetic material has been decreasing over time. How can the junk be decreasing? Surprisingly, the amount of junk has decreased to only 98.5% of genetic material. That is not a typo— less than 2% of the genetic material has a known function.[56] And so, once again, junk is just another term to simply our understanding. However, modern understanding of the cell and genetics is rapidly improving.

Returning to nicotine, its impact on bone formation and degradation is understood by the use of indirect markers in the blood and in bone. An indirect marker may indicate the presence of something that is difficult to detect in a direct manner. This is a common practice. "Direct markers" (an oxymoron) would be used if the technologies were well-developed. Indirect markers are analogous to looking for fingerprints. Except fingerprints are mostly unique; Scientific American suggests the odds of an identical set of fingerprints is one in 64 trillion. Unfortunately, indirect markers are much different than fingerprints. Similarities between markers lead to the very common issue where false positive findings result.

Suffice it to say, nicotine is associated with BMD, and variations in research methods lead to different results.

Does Switching to E-cigarettes and Vaping Help?

Before delving into the topic of E-cigarettes, or vaping, a brief history of tobacco use in the United States is important, as well as the introduction of the electronic cigarette. Smoking has actually declined from 20% of the population in 2014 to 14% of adults in 2019.[57]

Annual Prevalence of Smoking Among Adults > 18 Years, 2015-2019

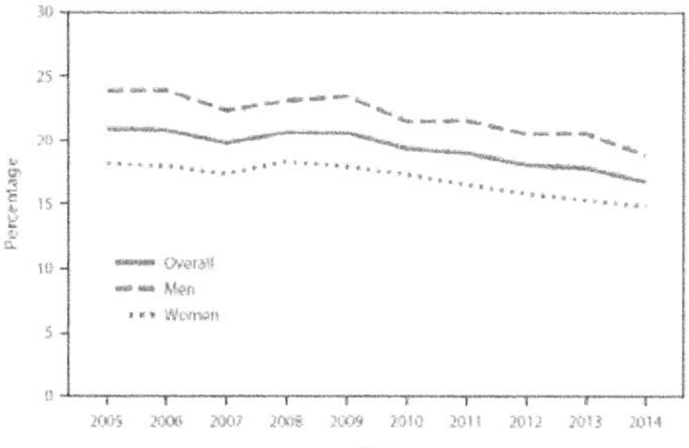

Figure 11. Prevalence of Smoking in Adults > 18. CDC Data.

The campaign against smoking and education regarding the negative health effects of smoking has also led to the decline in tobacco cigarette smoking in the United States. In the wake of a decline in tobacco smoking came the curious timing of electronic cigarette usage. After all, this is a technology that has been around, patented long ago. And yet, as smoking saw its decline, so did E-cigarettes see a simultaneous rise in popularity, which in 2011 was a 300% increase. How can one be sure exactly how many people switched from tobacco to E-cigarettes? Electronic cigarettes use a battery source to aerosolize a liquid pack containing nicotine and other chemicals. None of the chemicals have any reported health benefits. However, during the vaping process some chemicals can be formed as a product of the chemical reaction. The following correspondence in the prestigious *New England Journal of Medicine* where the researchers discuss all of the chemicals identified in e-cigarettes, none of which have been shown to have health benefits.

> "E-cigarette liquids are typically solutions of propylene glycol, glycerol, or both, plus nicotine and flavorant chemicals. We have observed that **formaldehyde-containing hemiacetals** ... can be formed during the e-cigarette "vaping" process. Formaldehyde is a known degradation product of propylene glycol that reacts with propylene glycol and glycerol during vaporization... **These molecules are known formaldehyde-releasing agents that are used as industrial biocides.**"[58] (emphasis added)

However, electronic cigarettes (ie., e-cigarettes, vaping) are marketed as a safer alternative to smoking.[59] Sadly, teen usage of e-cigarettes is skyrocketing. In one study of e-cigarette use among users aged 13 and 17, the main reason why e-cigarettes were preferred was due to the desirable flavor options.[60] Not only that, e-cigarettes are charged via USB, which potentially might interest a younger crowd (see figure below). E-cigarette usage certainly became convenient at the right time, when the "tobacco and cigarette" industry was seeing a decrease in use of tobacco. JUUL sales saw an increase by 14 million units in a single year between 2016 and 2017.

Select Examples of Electronic Cigarette Devices

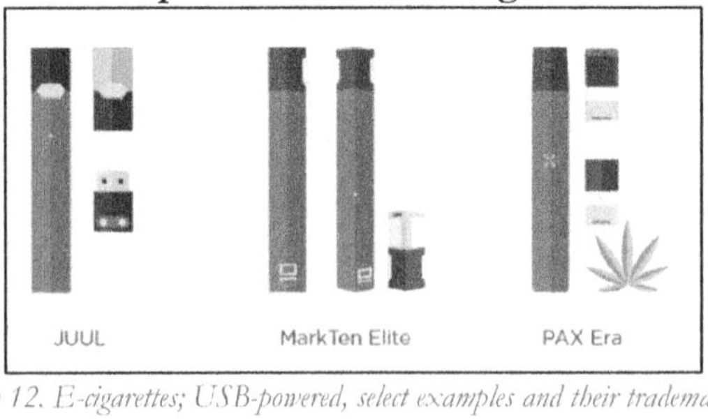

Figure 12. E-cigarettes; USB-powered, select examples and their trademarks.[61]

Making matters worse, the product JUUL (figure above, on left) contains the equivalent nicotine of 20 cigarettes in a single pod. There are differences between these products in terms of chemistry— work for the interested reader. However, how might someone without experience with smoking keep track of the amount of the pod they are taking in at once? One potential risk then is for the development of a rapid nicotine tolerance and addiction. As an aside, JUUL lost its first lawsuit in North Carolina pertaining to the claim of deceptive practices targeting teenagers. Overall, one can see how USB-powered cigarettes with flavors such as "Fruit Medley" and "Mango", and no way to keep track of nicotine intake may target a young crowd.[62]

The question arises about e-cigarette usage and bone density, which is an excellent question. There is actually laboratory research data that shows no significant adverse effect of E-vapor aerosols relative to tobacco cigarette exposure on bone density in mice.[63] Unfortunately, the conclusions that can be drawn from this study is that it is an animal model, where measurement of dose and response are improperly timed to show a negative result. In the case of some studies, authors employed by interested corporate parties is biased towards publishing only studies showing a benefit. In the case of the aforementioned laboratory study as well as many others, corporate funding is very common. It is very difficult to separate financial interests in these studies from objectivity.

Electronic cigarettes and Spinal Health

Ultimately, electronic cigarettes are relatively less well studied with regards to bone density and the spine. This is due to the young age of the product, and the young age of many of the users. In their review of e-cigarettes as it impacts spinal health, Fiani and coauthors highlight the impacts of chemical additives and the potential long term negative health risks of the spine.[64] However, there is no significant research that confirms this and therefore there are limitations in the study of e-cigarettes, which is what one would expect given that these products only gained popularity roughly 10 years ago.

Vitamins and Minerals and their Relationship with Osteoporosis

The most well studied aspect of diet is the relationship of vitamins and minerals and how they influence BMD.

Nutrition Nomenclature

Term	Definition
Micronutrient	A general term for vitamins and minerals.[65]
Water-soluble vitamins	Vitamin C, biotin, thiamin (B-1), riboflavin (B-2), niacin (B-3), pantothenic acid (B-5), pyridoxine (B-6), folic acid (B-9), cobalamin (B-12)
Fat-soluble vitamins	Vitamin A, D, E, K
Macro-minerals	Minerals where needs exceed 250 mg per day: Calcium, chloride, magnesium, phosphorus, potassium, sodium, and sulfur.
Trace minerals	Needs are below the 250 mg threshold: Chromium, copper, fluoride, iodine, iron, manganese, molybdenum, and zinc.

Table 1. Glossary of nutrient terms. For a list of updated daily recommended values, please see one example provided by the NIH Office of Dietary Supplements.

Calcium

Calcium is recommended for the prevention of osteoporosis, with a goal of 1,000 mg per day in adults. Supplementation with higher doses, up to 2100 mg per day, did not appear to provide a benefit in terms of increased BMD in either the hip or lumbar spine.[66] So there appears to be an upper limit of how much calcium is needed. Calcium will be discussed below in terms of nutrition, due to its importance.

Vitamin D and the "Calcium Paradox"

The work of American Biochemist Elmer McCollum led to his discovery of Vitamin A, B, and also Vitamin D. In collaboration with Edward Mellanby in 1919, he created a model for rickets development in rats and dogs, and demonstrated the treatment of this condition of low vitamin D, showing subsequent improvement with the consumption of cod liver oil. Cod liver oil is Vitamin D-rich.[67]

However, vitamin-D alone was only half of the story. Rickets had been well-known as a disease process since the 17th century in England when it was described by Francis Glisson, a disease which peaked during the period of rapid industrialization of Europe at the turn of the 20th century.[68] However, there was a missing piece to the puzzle. Exposure to sunlight and rapid improvement led to the experimental discovery of the relationship of Vitamin D and Rickets by Mellanby and McCollum. Ultimately, discovery of a more potent form of Vitamin D was discussed in *Rickets, Osteomalacia, and Tetany* by Hess in 1929:

> "The relationship of ergosterol to the etiology of rickets may be rationalized as follows: Ergosterol is contained in the skin and probably in almost all animal tissues and cells, in combination with the omnipresent cholesterol. In order to be activated, it requires but a small intensity of ultra-violet radiations and the resulting product is needed in but a minute fraction of a milligram to bring about calcification of the bones. **It is highly probable that the action of sunlight in protecting against rickets comes about through the mechanism of the activation of ergosterol in the skin and in its circulating blood.**"[69] (emphasis added)

Scientists have made significant progress in furtherance of our understanding of vitamin D and its activation by ultraviolet radiation from the sun at (at wavelengths 290-315 nanometers), which is enough energy to penetrate the outermost layer of our epidermis to "...convert 7-dehydrocholesterol (provitamin D3) to previtamin D3".[70] Once formed, pre-vitamin D3 slowly converts to the active form of vitamin D3 over 2-3 days. Interestingly enough, our skin pigment melanin, competes with provitamin D3 for ultraviolet radiation, and ultimately, individuals with darker skin require much longer sun exposure to develop the same amount of vitamin D3. Other impacts on the development of vitamin D3 includes one's age, sunscreen use, intensity of sunlight due to a number of environmental factors including latitude and duration of exposure, all of which impact the cutaneous production of vitamin D3.

For some time, scientists have been puzzled by the higher incidence of hip fractures in European and North American Societies where calcium is abundant in the diet. Meanwhile, in most of the developing world where there is less dietary calcium, hip fractures are less common. Without much additional information on the subject (such as genetics), one could hypothesize that increased dietary calcium causes fractures.

Anecdotally, for patients are against taking supplement formulations of calcium (eg. tablets), eggshells are almost entirely calcium. A medium egg has approximately 800 mg of elemental calcium. 40% of this is calcium carbonate is readily absorbable. But before abandoning this less than appealing idea, consider that most people pulverize the eggshell into a powder and mix with lemon juice, prior to consumption, a preparation that aids with taste. In a randomized, double-blind, placebo-controlled study over 1 year, women were randomized to either eggshell powder, alternative calcium carbonate vitamins, or placebo. Interestingly, only women in the group consuming eggshells saw an average increase in femoral neck bone density with decreases in markers for bone resorption.[2]

Perhaps Vitamin D may play an even greater importance than calcium. Some evidence suggests that calcium absorption and homeostasis is regulated by Vitamin D. Vitamin D has a recommended daily intake of 1300 IU per day. Studies of supplementation with Vitamin D in tandem with sources of calcium such as dairy products, suggests that the gains in BMD associated with milk, yogurt, and cheese were possibly due to, or dependent on Vitamin D supplementation.[71]

In the Boston Puerto Rico Osteoporosis Study, 904 people were surveyed, comprising 73% women, whereby total dairy intake and specific dairy products were itemized along with measurements of vitamin D levels. In the study, adequate vitamin D blood levels were defined as serum 25-hydroxyvitamin D $\geq$ 20 ng/mL. **What researchers observed was that having adequate vitamin D levels in tandem with increased dairy intake was associated with a higher BMD at the femoral neck and lumbar spine. If vitamin D levels were insufficient, increased dairy intake did not lead to a higher BMD.**[72] It is on the basis of many findings that calcium and vitamin D are both very important supplements, but it appears that inadequate vitamin D in its most active form, vitamin D3, has a relatively greater clinical impact on BMD between the two.

Acidic Foods

Apart from calcium and vitamin D content, due to the growth in popularity of the "health foods" market, more reports

---

[2] Increased calcium in the blood may indicate a net flow of calcium from the bones to the blood, a potential marker for resorption, among a number of other markers of resorption.

have questioned whether the acidity of what we eat and drink has an impact on BMD. If an acid is strong enough, it can breakdown substances over time. To use an (extreme) analogy, prior to coating a concrete surface, phosphoric acid is one liquid used to remove the superficial layer to allow a sealant to bind. That very same phosphoric acid is also contained in some sodas. As such, it is thought by many that phosphoric acid leaches calcium from teeth.

Chronic metabolic acidosis (relatively acidic blood), very commonly caused by chronic kidney disease, is a state of lowered pH below the physiologic range, and is associated with the progression of chronic kidney disease and osteoporosis.[73] In this acidosis, the blood comes nowhere near the level of acidity of the foods we eat, but nonetheless, a state of acidity is attained. The kidneys are a major mechanism for regulating pH in the blood,[74] and chronic untreated kidney disease can cause chronic acidosis. That is partially why dialysis is necessary in those with severely impaired or absent kidney function. So, the logic behind this concern stems from total of all acids ingested in the form of food and beverage in our diets— and whether this daily exposure to elevated acids in our foods and beverages can impact the development of osteoporosis.

It is important to define acidity as it pertains to human health. Acidity can be measured by pH, which goes by a scale of 0 to 14, where 0 is a pure acid and 14 is a pure base, and 7 is considered neutral, or a balanced acid and base state. For illustration purposes, battery acid has a pH of 0.5 and bleach has a pH of 12.5, which are mentioned for reference— avoid contact between those two. As we see, the further away from neutral (7), and the closer to a pure acid or pure base, the more caustic these substances. The pH of normal biological processes is 7.36 to 7.44 and the pH within the cell is estimated at 7.2. The presence of special molecules in the blood called buffers help maintain the pH between the aforementioned range by binding to excess acids or bases. In the case of the blood, examples of buffers are carbonic acid and hydrogen carbonate. In a chronic acidosis, bone is a major source of pH buffer, in the form of calcium carbonate. The reaction releases calcium, and that is one manner in which calcium can leave the bone. The body is never this simple, but the important point here is that the body is a brilliant system with numerous mechanisms to keep the body running optimally.

Influence of Diet Choices on BMD

Independent of Vitamin D and Calcium, and other vitamins and minerals, adequate calorie and protein intake may impact BMD. So, it is not just vitamins and minerals, but potentially other nutrition that is required. The challenge is identifying cause and effect, and not misreading a correlation. For example, Qing and coinvestigators studied the potential impact of a diet high in meat intake across 1905 study participants, finding meat to be protective for the development of osteoporosis[75], as well as the consumption of fish.[76] That is of course not surprising, since these animals have bones, and you would expect to find them full of substances that support the development of bone. In this regard, more work needs to be done.

Isoflavones, a class of phytoestrogens, are a type of soy protein found in plants. Their estrogenic property is said to be protective of the loss of BMD. Chinese researchers similarly looked at a representative sample of 454 women within the first 12 years of menopause, confirming the suspected positive relationship with increased soy intake and improved BMD and bone mineralization.[77] Interestingly in a large cross-sectional study of one community, osteoporosis was found to be more common in women who favored a diet of vegetables over any kind of fish or meat.[78] The reader must keep in mind that the questionnaire did not study what kind of vegetables to assess for relevant nutrients and other lifestyles. Again, a study like this will certainly highlight interesting areas of further research, but exhaustive study of other variables that can influence the results needs to be done before conclusions may be drawn.

The Relationship Between Dairy Products and Bone Health

Obviously, the health benefits of milk needs no introduction. Generally, most people would not object to the widespread belief that drinking milk results in healthy bones. In fact, in the 2018 article, "Dairy Products and Bone Health: How Strong is the Evidence?", the authors feel that the matter is settled:

> "In conclusion, the role of dairy products for BMC or BMD has been sufficiently established in Chinese and Caucasian girls and women. In Caucasian women, drinking milk also reduces fracture risk. More research on the role of dairy products within the context of bone health-promoting diets is needed in specific ethnicities, other than Chinese and Caucasians, and in men."[79]

How about drinking half and half, is that good for bones? Or, how about cheese, yogurt, or any other dairy product? Are they good for the bones? Believe it or not, these food products have been studied at one point or another to answer this question.

Milk is the most well-studied dairy product in terms of bone health. Again, one frequently quoted study is the Framingham Study, which will be able to provide some insight. In the initial 1988 population of patients, 980 patients were surveyed in a 2008 follow-up, and it was noted that milk consumption was associated with a 43% reduction in hip fracture.[80] Another study conducted in Northern Italy of 241 postmenopausal women over the age of 45 who had a hip fracture, as compared with 719 controls, found no appreciable benefit of milk. This fracture risk did not appear to change, regardless of the amount of milk consumption.[81]

Perhaps the effects of milk are insignificant next to the impact of the changes that occur due to hormone deficiency in menopause? In one cross-sectional study, milk consumption did not appear to improve BMD in women, but it did appear to improve BMD in men. Meanwhile, calcium supplementation was associated with increased BMD in all groups.[82]

The authors could not observe a lower likelihood of fracture, regardless of frequency and total amount of milk, cheese, or overall calcium intake. These are puzzling results. Sometimes, when there are multiple studies with conflicting results, a type of study called a meta-analysis is turned to, which might be able to provide further insight. A meta-analysis uses statistics to aggregate the findings. One chief flaw is that it is not a study on its own, and it repurposes data from dissimilar studies. If 20 studies with flawed methodology all reach flawed conclusions, aggregating their results will merely summarize flawed findings.

Nonetheless, a meta-analysis conducted to summarize the results of 18 studies aimed to find a relationship between dairy consumption and hip fracture risk. Unfortunately, the authors were unable to find that milk consumption led to a reduction in hip fractures.[83] However, when looking at yogurt and cheese consumption, a reduction in hip fractures was observed and a significant improvement in BMD was observed in the greater trochanter and lumbar spine (See table below).

In looking at the table, cream was observed to have a decreased bone density in all groups, but those changes were slight and were not statistically significant.

Cheese and Bone Mineral Density

In the aforementioned Framingham Study, yogurt appeared to have the only significant impact on BMD, and cheese had a nonsignificant trend towards lower BMD in postmenopausal women. Cheese may still have some benefit, particularly in adolescent girls, however. In one study of ten to twelve year-old girls, dietary calcium intake was assessed among four groups: I: 200 mg calcium + vitamin D3 (200 IU), II: 1000 mg Calcium supplements, III: cheese (estimated 1000 mg Calcium), and IV: placebo (no supplementation). Results of bone densitometry testing performed at the conclusion of the study showed a significantly greater cortical bone thickness and superior BMD at all measured sites throughout the body.[84] Cheese appears to have a greater impact on BMD than other dairy products, perhaps due to its high nutrient density— it contains plenty of fat, protein, calcium, vitamin D, antioxidant and probiotics byproducts of fermentation are potentially helpful as well.

Probiotics and prebiotics are food containing live microorganisms and food intended to support this flora, respectively. Recent popularity in probiotics is a curious thing, as many of these products are relatively expensive. Probiotics are abundant in fermented foods, and some fermented foods like, beer, cheese, and wine, and are over 10,000 years old.[80] Cheese is not a simple process, and the people that discovered this likely observed the benefits. Eleven cheeses are probiotic: Feta, Swiss, Gouda, Edam, Caciocavallo, Emmental, Gruyere, Cottage, Parmesan, Provolone, and Raw Cheddar. Results from several studies show probiotics are associated with improved BMD.[85]

Association Between Dairy Product Consumption and Hip Fracture Development: Framingham Study

Dairy Exposure	BMD (Femoral Neck)	BMD (Trochanter)	BMD (Lumbar Spine)
Milk	+, NS	+, NS	+, NS
Yogurt (≤4 servings/week)	-, NS	-, NS	-, NS
Yogurt (>4 servings/week)	+, NS	+	+
Cheese (2-4 servings/week)	+, NS	-, NS	-, NS
Cheese (>4 servings/week)	+, NS	+, NS	**+, NS**
Cream	-, NS	-, NS	-, NS

Table 2 Association Between Dairy Product Consumption and Hip Fracture Development: Results of the Framingham Osteoporosis Study. Statistically significant results are shaded, and observed only in yogurt consumption greater than 4 servings per week, where there was an increase in BMD in the trochanteric femur and lumbar spine. NS – not significant. +/- denotes a respective increase or decrease in final BMD.

Vitamin D in Dairy Products in the Prevention of Osteoporosis

Vitamin D is thought to be an essential component in supplementation for the prevention of Osteoporosis. What is the relative benefit of supplementation versus obtaining this vitamin from dairy sources? Unfortunately, what can be shown at the least is that vitamin D is helpful. For the benefit of the additional nutrients contained in the whole foods that contain vitamin D, it is advisable, whenever possible, to obtain as much vitamins and minerals from a healthy diet, without a reliance upon supplementation. According to the National Institute of

Health (NIH), one gram of calcium and 4,000 IU daily[3] of Vitamin D are recommended for adults.[86]

Beverages and Their Impact on BMD

So, can foods and drinks overwhelm the acid-base system? What is the pH of our food and beverages? Many of the beverages we drink are surprisingly acidic. A few beverages have been illustrated in the table below. Acidic beverages have been demonstrated to be a determinant of dental erosion caused by acids such as phosphoric and citric acids. This is in itself argued as evidence of the plausibility that acidic beverages could potentially erode bone.[87] However, for this to be true, it is assumed that the acids are not neutralized by a base, which is improbable.

---

[3] The term IU refers to international unit, and is generally used to refer to the measurement of fat-soluble vitamins only. The conversion of IU to mg is specific to each fat-soluble vitamin, which are vitamins A, D, E, and K.

Common Acidic Beverages and Their pH Values‡

Beverage	**pH**
Lemon Juice	2.25
Coca-Cola Classic®	2.34
Coca-Cola Caffeine Free ®	2.38
Pepsi ®	2.39
Gatorade® Lemon-Lime	2.75
Arizone Iced Tea	2.85
Coca-Cola Zero ®	2.96
Gatorade® Orange	2.99
Coca-Cola Diet ®	3.10
Mountain Dew®	3.22
Pineapple Juice (Dole ®)	3.40
Redbull Regular ®	3.43
Apple Juice (Tropicana ®)	3.50
Orange Juice (Tropicana ®)	3.80
Tomato Juice (Campbell ®)	4.01
Water (Dasani®)	5.03
Starbucks Medium Roast®	5.11
Water (Aquafina®)	6.11

‡- *General abbreviated table of common beverages and their average pH values as sourced from a publication of the American Dental Association in 2016.*[88]

Fruits and vegetables display a somewhat greater variability in pH ranging from 2.00 for limes to 7.50 for olives.[88] Ethanol, found in alcoholic beverages, have a pH close to neutral, with a pH of 7.33. The process of fermentation that makes alcoholic beverages, generates acid byproducts, and in one study of different beers, a pH range between 4.3 and 4.55 may be found.[89] The pH of wine did not differ dramatically and the author did not consider the thousands of specialty beverages. One last word regarding these food and beverage pH values. They vary considerably. The value for green tea may be reported to vary from 6.5 to 10![90] Also, consider that the pH of water varies and can cause variability, when considering beverages that are not regulated by a standardized manufacturing processes (eg. industrial beverages such as colas and beer that use their own water purification process). What does that mean for our overall health? Frankly, that is not well understood.

Therefore, the question arises as to whether or not a diet high in acidic foods and beverages could lead to bone loss, of which there is data in favor of, and against this presupposition. Acidic foods are neutralized by an alkalinic (basic) salt well before influencing the pH of our blood, where life is only supported between a narrow range of neutral values. The activity of the acid on the bone is indirect. Demineralization of the teeth is thought to occur directly with a pH below 5.5. That is the issue with direct contact of liquids. Thankfully, your bones are not being washed directly by these caustic beverages.

Studies of the mineralization of bone shows that bone contains a large reservoir of these alkaline compounds, which would aid in the neutralization of increased concentrations of acids.[91] Since pH regulation is absolutely vital to life, the body makes use of chemical buffers that help maintain a range of pH values. The bone is one such reservoir of buffer in that manner that dissolved limestone can buffer acid rain— an example of the macrocosm and the microcosm.

Do Carbonated Beverages Cause Osteoporosis?

Carbonated beverages include sodas, seltzer water, and sparkling mineral water. Another common belief is that these beverages negatively impact osteoporosis. Perhaps the largest clinical study evaluating dietary measures and osteoporosis development was again found in the Framingham Osteoporosis Study. This study measured spine and hip BMD in 1413 women and 1125 men and evaluated food consumption by questionnaire. Only a correlation between carbonated cola beverages and osteoporosis was found, and not among non-cola carbonated beverages. Perhaps it was not the carbonation, but the phosphoric acid contained in cola, as the active agent. This correlation was found in older women, and not in men.[92] It is important to keep that, relative to women, men are less prone to osteoporosis in older ages. This association in women is not a definitive finding due to limitations in the study design. Due to the recognized study limitations, the authors did not conclude that carbonated cola beverages cause osteoporosis.

Also, numerous risk factors can impact the results, regardless of the size of the study population. The use of a survey may introduce additional bias as the data being collected is at the mercy of the recollection of the interviewee. Hence, the accuracy of the data becomes unknown to the principle investigator. There are numerous ways that bias and error can be introduced into a study this way. For a more complete understanding of the challenges of research conducted in this manner, the author recommends the book, *Internet, Phone, and Mixed-mode Surveys: The Tailored Design Method* which provides an excellent insight into how these types of studies are conducted so provide the highest quality study possible.[93]

Does Protein Intake Impact Osteoporosis?

Low protein intake has been associated with osteoporosis development. However, one challenge to studying this is the issue of malnourished individuals being depleted in vitamins and minerals as well as protein. This confounding issue is most often attempted to be solved with the use of statistical tests. Unfortunately, this can be problematic as the choice of statistical test to use can vary among statisticians, as there are many options, and some forms of statistical testing may be thought to be superior to another. For a very thoughtful review of the problems with significance testing, the author recommends the article, "Use, Overuse, and Misuse of Significance Tests in Evolutionary Biology and Ecology."[94]

Does Caffeine Consumption Impact Osteoporosis?

Caffeine has become an essential part in American lives. In America, over 54% of adults over 18 are said to consume caffeine every day.[95] In a survey of the US Department of Agriculture study between 1994 and 1998 the most common sources of caffeine in beverages were coffee, soft drinks, and tea in 71, 16, and 12% of adults, respectively.[96] The FDA has recommended that healthy adults should limit their intake to 400 mg per day, which they estimate at 4 or 5 standardized cups of coffee per day. However, as most people are aware, the body metabolizes caffeine fairly rapidly, and toxic effects of excessive caffeine, such as seizures, do not manifest until about 1200 mg of caffeine are very rapidly consumed in a short time.[97]

Metabolic Effects of Caffeine

The metabolic effects of caffeine are extensive and only a few aspects need be discussed in order to gain a better sense of the impact of caffeine on bone metabolism. First, caffeine has been associated with decreased absorption of calcium and increased urinary excretion of calcium. Laboratory evidence suggests caffeine could potentially influence the normal physiologic binding site of the vitamin D receptors, negatively impairing bone development. While it seems that caffeine may not be of any benefit, there is some very curious evidence produced in the past several years that is contrary to these claims.

Caffeine and the Bone Growth, Density, and Height

Most of the studies on caffeine effects are studied in adults, and due to the wide-ranging effects of caffeine on the growing adolescent, this aspect will be omitted. Adults comprise the majority of people with osteoporosis and they will be the focus. However, briefly, has the reader ever heard someone say that a child or adolescent should not have any caffeine-containing drinks, because it will "stunt their growth"? Well, there is evidence of the association between caffeine consumption and bone growth impairment. In animal studies, Choi and coinvestigators provide evidence in their rat study that caffeine adversely impacts numerous metabolic pathways, contributing to the decreased longitudinal bone growth.[98] Longitudinal bone growth is what occurs in long bones of our extremities and contributes to our final height. The authors also found a negative impact on chondrocytes, which serve a few roles, such as in cartilage development, but are also present in the growth plates of the growing adolescent. In another animal study, rats in the high dose caffeine group were noted to have a significantly shorter and less dense tibia, femur, and vertebral column.[99] Let's keep in mind that critics of these types of experimentation rightly argue that maintaining and understanding chemical concentrations in small mammals is difficult. Do these studies represent a realistic doses encountered in humans? Often, the dose may be too high.[100] In another rat study, rats were divided into four groups: exercise only, caffeine and no exercise, both caffeine and exercise, and a control group (neither caffeine nor exercise). The authors found that "...caffeine feeding decreased the weight and total calcium content of the femur." Any yet, high doses of caffeine appeared to stimulate the growth of long bone..."[100] Exercise did not appear to mitigate the effects of caffeine and that avoidance of caffeine was the best way to limit the extent of this impact. The authors found that the negative effects outweighed the positive effects in this study citing a net bone mineral loss, lower BMD, and decreased calcium content. However, at the same time, high dose caffeine had the opposite effect of the relatively lower dose group, which is paradoxical and no plausible explanation may be offered.

Clinical Studies of Caffeine Use and Bone Density

The increase in total amount of daily caffeine has been reported to be related to a decrease in BMD in day. However, this does not say that caffeine causes osteoporosis. This can be understood in one of the following ways. Perhaps it depends on the beverage. If participants in the studies are followed for a limited time, as they usually are studied for some duration less than five years, their T-score will not often drop from above 0 to below -2.5, in such a short time, with some less common exceptions. And for patients in one group with borderline osteopenia, lets say for example, -2.49, and five years later then have -2.55 and are now given a diagnosis of osteoporosis, does that mean that their respective exposures to daily caffeine consumption were the cause of this diagnosis of osteoporosis? Most likely not, but impossible to show.

Small changes in many co-dependent variables being studied in an ocean of unknown variables must be understood for what they are, which is that that the significance is unknown. A "significant" change in BMD is dependent on the chosen statistical test, in many cases. Often, relative rates and relative measures and significance are the only reported results and there is much less raw data to compare.

In the Nord-Trøndelag Health Survey, 1652 randomly selected perimenopausal and postmenopausal Norweigian women were assessed for risk factors that develop osteoporosis. In the analysis of the results, using statistical modeling to account for multiple variables (a multivariate model), both the pack-years of smoking[4] and daily coffee intake was observed to have a negative impact on the BMD of the distal radius (near the wrist) alone.[101]

---

[4] This is how healthcare professionals and scientists measure the product of number of cigarettes each day and number of years of use in a single measure. For example, "10 pack-years" can mean anything ranging from one pack per day for ten years or even to half a pack per day for 20 years. They are multiplied together to reach the measure of ten pack-years.

With the complexities of clinical studies in mind, there are a number of interesting studies assessing BMD, fracture, and the exposure to caffeine, or caffeine-containing beverages such as coffee and tea, with further assessment as to the amount of cups per day. The prevailing public opinion seems to be that caffeine consumption leads to a deterioration in the bones. And to support that, in adult women with over 300 mg/day of daily caffeine intake, accelerated BMD loss was reported.[102]

While there are human clinical studies as well that provide evidence of the ill-effects of caffeine on osteoporosis, one large study in the USA, again, the Framingham Osteoporosis Study, did not find a relationship between caffeine intake and decreased BMD, while simultaneously finding a relationship between smoking and decreased BMD.[103] In contrast, a study of 1817 Chinese menopausal women found coffee consumption to be an independent and significant risk for the development osteoporosis, not just a decrease in BMD.[51]

Since the most common caffeinated products that are consumed are either carbonated as in sodas or acidic, one can reasonably deduce that an impact would be detected for both the reasons of acidity and the content of caffeine. However, the study found an association between cola and decreased BMD, which is carbonated. Therefore, one would think that there is a contradiction. However, if one spends enough time evaluating longitudinal studies of large groups of people where data is gathered over time, seemingly contradictory or unexplained findings do occur. This highlights the difficulty with studying the multifactorial process of osteoporosis that takes a long time to develop. One often overlooked aspect in this study, and most others is the presence of genetic risk factors for osteoporosis development. That is because genetic risk factors are not completely well understood.

Coffee Intake and Fracture Risk

One consideration is that coffee contains another chemical other than caffeine that may have an impact on bone physiology or calcium regulation, or other related pathways, and that this potential unidentified substance could be accounting for the majority of the findings. This hypothesis is possibly supported by one study of liver cirrhosis, which found that coffee consumption, but not other caffeine containing beverages such as soda, was potentially inhibiting the onset of alcoholic and non-alcoholic liver cirrhosis.[104] One may ask themselves how a liver study and an entirely different patient population serves useful evidence to the study of bone regulation, caffeine, and the development of osteoporosis. The answer is that a cup of coffee may contain more than just caffeine that is physiologically active.

Previous human clinical studies find challenges with monitoring caffeine. There were several metabolites of caffeine that can be tracked. A metabolite is a product of breakdown of the parent chemical, and still biologically active. For example, nicotine is inactivated by the enzyme CYP2A6 to cotinine and then to 3'hydroxycotinine.[105] Some metabolites persist in the body for a longer duration than others, and some metabolites have a relatively greater physiologic effect.

Very High Coffee Intake- Is it Protective?

While negative effects of caffeine on bone have been demonstrated in the aforementioned laboratory studies, conflicting evidence exists in some large clinical studies, highlighting a possible protective effect at the upper limits of the population curve, in terms of daily caffeine intake. In the Hong Kong Osteoporosis Study, two groups totaling 564 people were studied, finding 12 metabolites associated with coffee consumption, and 6 that were associated with caffeine.[106] The authors found increased bone density at the spine and femoral neck in coffee drinkers, which conflicts with the above studies.

Perhaps further studies are necessary to determine what the significance, if any, of these metabolites serve for researching the complex relationship of osteoporosis and caffeine consumption. In the Korean National Health and Nutrition Examination Survey conducted from 2008-2011, 4066 postmenopausal women were assessed over time, using a representative sample of the general Korean population of women with a mean age of 62 years. Researchers found very interesting results. The authors observed that coffee consumption may be protective in patients in the highest coffee consumption group.[107]

The aim of caffeine on hip fracture risk was studied. In Italian women, 279 women with hip fractures were compared to 1061 women with matched characteristics. The authors did not find any relationship between coffee consumption, or any other caffeine-containing beverage and a risk for having a hip fracture. Interestingly, they could not find a risk for hip fracture, regardless of the frequency of coffee consumption, and among their sample of patients, they were able to have sufficient numbers to study patients by the number of cups per day. Overall, no difference in risk for hip fracture was found, regardless of the number of cups of coffee per day, even up to the upper limit of 5 cups per day.[108] Overall, a meta-analysis of twelve studies containing data on coffee consumption and hip fractures found no significant relationship between coffee consumption and hip fracture development.[109]

Tea Consumption and Hip Fracture Risk

Since there are many people that drink tea instead of coffee, it would not be fair to ignore the well-studied relationship between tea consumption and coffee. A meta-analysis summarized the results of 9 studies, totaling 147, 950 patients, which found no significant association between tea consumption and preventing fracture development.[110] In other words, no evidence of benefit or harm was observed. And yet, in a large meta-analysis including 16 studies, including an impressive 772,707 patients, of which there were 37,166 fractures observed, the authors found a slight beneficial and hence protective effect of tea consumption on fracture formation.[111] Again, always keep in mind that these meta-analyses are synthesizing different studies to find a risk reduction in fractures, and not a reduction in BMD. It would be expected that researchers would have a harder time showing a greater improvement in BMD needed to prevent fractures than showing a significant improvement in BMD alone.

Some of the authors note the numerous limitations of studying tea consumption including data collection challenges and the significant variation in the herbs and other additives to tea which limits the ability to synthesize the results of multiple studies. After all, everyone's definition of tea isn't the same, just the same as with coffee, and different species of plant can have different physiologically active compounds.

The Unique Properties of Green Tea and Impact on Bone Density

Green tea is thought to be beneficial for general health. Is it helpful for improving BMD? A study of the green tea composition found that more than 80% of green tea polyphenols are catechins.[112] It is incredible how extensively researched catechins are as an anti-inflammatory molecule. In bone, catechins have been shown to regulate the RANK/RANKL/OPG pathway in osteoblast cells[113] Published in the journal *Antioxidants,* is the article titled, "Osteoprotective Roles of Green Tea Catechins", whereby Huang and co-authors discuss the beneficial impact of green tea catechins on bone health.[114] Studies of catechin effects have often shown a significant improvement in BMD.

Exercise and Osteoporosis

There are numerous health benefits of exercise, and it is basically a common assumption that exercise is helpful for preventing a decrease in bone density. This is a lot harder to consistently demonstrate in studies. After all, exercise is a subjective term.

By now, the reader probably is not surprised that studying exercise and demonstrating positive benefits in a scientific manner is more challenging than it seems. For example, just looking at 12 members of a track team and comparing them to 12 professional bowling "athletes" seems like a great way to prove a difference. But then a lot of different variables must be taken into consideration. Perhaps the diets are different and some of the "athletes" smoke, all of which could prevent any meaningful answers from being obtained.

When patients discuss their exercise, often the point comes up that they walk a certain number of miles, ergo, they exercise. But what is the definition of exercise in terms of exertion level and duration, if any? Also, exercise is not just aerobic activity—"Harvard Health Publishers" lists 4 classes of exercise. These are important in maintaining wellness. They include aerobic exercise (cardiovascular/ "cardio"), such as walking, running, swimming, and biking, weight-training, stretching, and balance exercises. All of these are advocated as needing to be incorporated into an exercise routine.[115] So, in general, everyone considers exercise differently, and relevant exercise differs depending on what the benefit one wants to achieve. Blood pressure reduction usually is associated with more rigorous exercise schedules.

Laboratory Animal Studies: Exercises and Bone Density

Laboratory exercise studies are difficult to extrapolate to human results, but often provide meaningful information nonetheless. For example, one rat study of exercise amounted to one mile divided over one hour, daily, for five days per week for wither seven weeks or eleven weeks, with control comparisons to rats having not had exercise activity. Again, rather than try to understand this study design, extrapolating this to humans is the real challenge. For one, estimates of regular walking pace (moderate) are to three miles per hour, and exertion level is not known. Overall, the authors found that treadmill exercise stimulated the formation of bone and the suppression of bone resorption.[116] Moreover, an increase in 1,25-dihydroxyvitamin D-(3) in the blood and decrease in the parathyroid hormone level was also measured. Overall, these are all good observations, and an increased measure of bone mass was observed in young growing rats, which were measurably larger.

Clinical Studies of Exercise and Impact on Bone Density

As explained in the preceding section, to gain a sufficient insight into research in this topic, for someone who has no experience in laboratory animal research—exercise intensity and duration are key components in understanding if there are to be any health benefits of exercise. This leads to the question as to whether or not exercise improves bone density or in other words is preventative in the development of osteoporosis. Just keep in mind that even if certain exercises were studied and no significant impact on osteoporosis was demonstrated, just as with quitting smoking, there are numerous benefits to exercise and perhaps these secondary effects may improve BMD in addition to quality of life.

Human clinical studies have found largely benefits to exercise for BMD. In one randomized clinical trial in Germany, 227 women were randomized to a higher intensity exercise group, or the control group, being a low intensity "wellness" program. The study lasted approximately 18 months. Researchers found significant benefits of exercise on BMD, and a reduced number of falls.[117] In another study of 160 osteopenic women, a home-based exercise program of lower intensity was evaluated across seven years. In this study, a reduction in overall fractures was found. [118] In a much longer follow-up of 16 years, 105 German women were surveyed in the Erlangen Fitness and Osteoporosis Prevention Study.[119] Overall, exercise was associated with a significantly lower overall fracture risk. In these studies, fairly consistent benefit was shown for exercise on bone density.

The question as to whether or not there is a benefit to a regular exercise routine on bone health and increasing BMD may seem obvious now, but the answer is surprising— There are studies that suggest it is helpful, and others that suggest there is no benefit. There is no way to reconcile this.

For example, surprisingly, The Framingham Osteoporosis Study did not demonstrate a significant relationship between exercise and BMD.[120] In one review of the subject of osteoporosis and exercise, one medical researcher concludes that, "Moderate exercise protects against osteoporosis, but too little or excessive exercise may cause osteoporosis."[51] Keep in mind that little, moderate, or excessive exercise are poorly defined terms. Still, there are a number of studies demonstrating a positive benefit of exercise and the general health effects of exercise cannot be overlooked. However, the idea of excessive exercise having negative consequences on bone health sounds intuitive, as this can cause repetitive micro-injury of the bone and deplete stores of calcium.

Excessive Exercise and Bone Density

"Excessive" exercise, is an ill-defined term, and is a term often encountered in studies of athletes. Loss of BMD in excessive exercise is thought to result from decreased levels of sex hormones observed in endurance athletes. Perhaps also, the calcium needs of athletes are greater than most, as all muscle cells utilize calcium ions as their main intracellular signaling molecule. The strength of a muscle contraction is dependent on proteins involved in calcium signaling.[121] Calcium storage and release is related to muscle fatigue and cramping.[122] Perhaps also, it is not excessive physical demand and stress. This finding of loss of bone density as a result of decreased sex hormones in the endurance athlete was similarly concluded by Voss and coauthors and published in the *Journal of the American Academy of Orthopedics.*[122]

Amenorrhea, which is the absence of menstruation, implies chronic hypoestrogenism when studied in young female athletes. In studying this population of women, scientists suggest that inadequate caloric intake in tandem with chronic high caloric demands of exercise leads to bone loss.[123] Perhaps also, the simple negative calorie balance over a prolonged time period can result in catabolism — ie. not just the loss of fat, but the loss of muscle and bone as well.

6 Screening

Often, osteoporosis is identified at two time points: late, and much too late. Screening of patients over 50 helps to identify the estimate 20% of men and at least 37% of women who have a significant loss of bone density, and are said to be in need of preventative treatment.[124]

Patients are identified either before or after a fracture, many of which are debilitating or life-threatening. A common scenario of a fracture comes from a "slip and fall", a manner that is often surprising. For example, slipping in the bathtub. Diagnosis of osteoporosis comes through screening bone densitometry, and should occur, *before* the fracture. Screening assists with the prevention of fractures. Deterioration of bone density is insidious, and can reach significant levels in up to one-sixth of the US population without a single warning sign. There are no warning signs, apart from the diligent healthcare providers warning the patient to get screened. Perhaps with screening, once identified, the clinical course could be reversed through lifestyle modification, avoidance of certain activities, quitting smoking, and ensuring enough calcium and vitamin D3 intake in order to limit bone breakdown and facilitate bone development.

The importance of screening for osteoporosis has been established by the fact that multiple societies have produced fairly updated guidelines. These reports have been issued by the American Association of Family Practicioners[125,126], American Society of Endocrinologists,[127,128] American College of Rheumatology,[129] American College of Physicians,[130] as well as European Societies.[131,132] Tables for the Abbreviated major risk factors and screening recommendations are provided below.

Risk Factors for Osteoporosis[5]

Parental History of Hip Fracture
Excess alcohol consumption
Smoking
Low Body Weight

Screening Recommendations for The Prevention of Osteoporotic Compression Fractures

Women 65 years or older
Postmenopausal Women of any age

FRAX®: The Fracture Risk Assessment Tool

[5] Not a comprehensive list. For a more complete list, which includes numerous medications, please see the section on risk factors.

There are measurement systems to give people a general idea of their risk for an osteoporotic fracture. These are provided in no definite terms, as all studies are comprised of unique individuals with unique lifestyles, environmental exposures, and risk factors such as age, medication use, and medical history. All of these factors can result in an increased risk for osteoporosis.

One tool, The Fracture Risk Assessment Tool, or FRAX®, developed by the Center for Metabolic Bone Diseases at Sheffield University, gives a 10 year probability of hip fracture and major osteoporotic fracture such as spine, forearm, hip, or shoulder.[6] Keep in mind that the developers of FRAX® use a 10 year-probability provide number that is, "...more readily understood by patients"[133], which is to say, provide a larger number that will "prompt" (scare) a patient to participate in the recommended preventative care of osteoporosis.

FRAX® Estimates Of 10-Year Probability Of A Major Osteoporotic Fracture[134]

Age Group (years)	Mean Probability (%)
40-49	2.59
50-59	5.54
60-69	7.77
70-79	9.57
80 and over	11.35

Obesity – Stress Fractures – and Osteoporosis Correlation in The Adolescent

Osteoporosis is not unheard of, even in seemingly healthy young adults. While it is uncommon, the growing prevalance of obesity in adolescents makes this topic worthy of discussion as

[6] For Personal review of one's risk, as of 2021, this can be accessed at: https://www.sheffield.ac.uk/FRAX/reference.aspx

it gives further insight into the disease. The percent of obese and extremely obese have shown a dramatic increase since 1960 (see figure below). There have been numerous detrimental changes in the adolescent diet and lifestyle compared to 50 years ago. Books written for the general public and dedicated to the study of the "obesity epidemic" can be purchased at a local bookstore. For example, *The Obesity Epidemic* by Zoe Harcombe and numerous other provocative titles go in depth on the societal problems and task of combatting obesity.

Obesity in the United States, 1969-2008

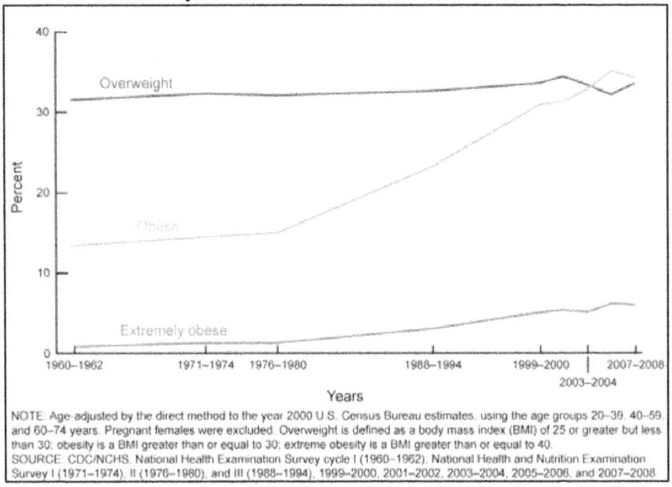

Figure 13. CDC: Prevalence of Overweight, Obesity, and Extreme Obesity Among Adults: United States, Trends 1960–1962, Through 2007–2008[135]

While osteoporotic fractures of the spine are very rare in teenagers and young adults of generations past and present, a study of this special population over time may suggest that bone quality is deteriorating for this group. In the 18 year-old, military cadet, stress fractures have become a growing problem, particularly femoral neck and tibial fractures. And while the military cadet is a very niche group that is not representative of the population, it is a well-studied group who are representative sample of the general population at the start of the study. The hypothesis is that these extreme demands of weight-bearing and fatigue required of a female cadet are beyond the strength of the bone, which therefore must be deteriorating, if we assume that the bone quality of the female of the cadet is representative of the general 18 year-old population, and deteriorating. The stress fractures encountered in the young female soldier are femoral neck fractures.

This can be compared to the distribution of fractures in the fifty year-old population. The figure below shows the prevalence of both low bone mass and osteoporosis both in the femoral neck and the lumbar spine.

Prevalence and Extent of Osteoporosis, and Low Bone Mass

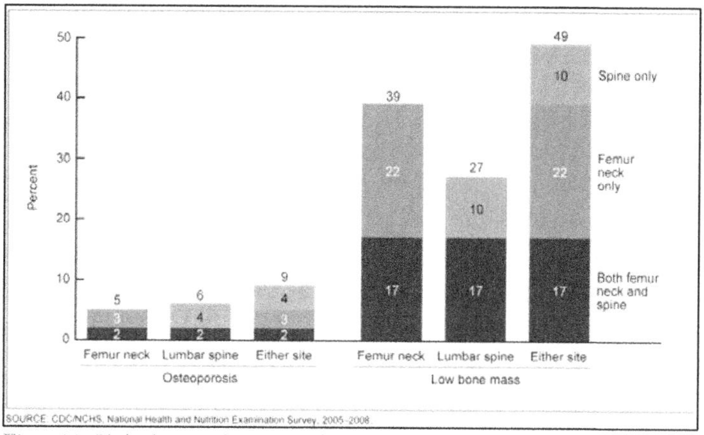

Figure 14 Skeletal status of persons aged 50 years and over: United States, 2005-2008. (source:CDC/NCHS, National Health and Nutrition Survey, 2005-2008). .[136]

There appears to be a higher proportion of femoral neck fractures in 18 year-old female cadets than the general osteoporosis population. Perhaps it is due to deteriorating nutrition, by way of high calorie, nutrient-poor[7] foods resulting

---

[7] To illustrate nutrient density- soda and a cup of orange juice have similar calories and similar sugar, depending on the source, whereas orange juice has vitamin C, making it more nutrient dense.

in chronic vitamin deficiency. It is easily provable that our food is deteriorating for a variety of reasons. But that is not the only proposed mechanism of adolescent stress fractures. Numerous other causes proposed range from the increasingly sedentary lifestyle, increased consumption of fast food, alterations in the genetics of the food supply, reliance on technology for entertainment and transportation over exercise means, and decreased reliance on manual labor in general.

Returning to the discussion of adolescent stress fractures. In general, army clinicians calculated an 8.5% risk of stress fracture every 8 weeks of basic training for women, slightly higher than in men. When one thinks about it, that is a very significant number! But, what is the link between a stress fracture and osteoporosis? It would be misleading to say that osteoporosis was present and the primary cause of these fractures in someone's "peak years". And yet, the risk factors in these young athletic populations, closely match risk factors later in life. So, osteoporotic risk factors are the same as those risk factors for stress fracture early in life.[137] As alluded to previously, one of the biggest issues with these studies is that we have not bridged the gap required to study "bone microarchitecture", which is thought to be just as important as BMD. And if the architecture of the bone cannot be studied, and the BMD does not change appreciably, then this leads to difficulties with elaborating the causes of fracture.

While definitive causality has not been demonstrated, early interventions to treat risk factors for stress fractures have led to a lower risk of stress fracture for female cadets. These modifications in lifestyle, diet, and in the following military study, calcium and vitamin D supplementation, have been linked with less stress fractures in female navy recruits. Lappe and coinvestigators randomized 5201 female navy recruits in this double blinded, placebo-controlled study to 2000mg Calcium and 800 IU Vitamin D or placebo.[138] In this study, the overall incidence of stress fractures were 5.9% every 8 weeks, and 20% lower in the group with supplementation. Of the 14,416 women who entered basic training over two years, they estimate that 187 women would have been able to have avoided a fracture.

Obesity- A Major Healthcare Issue – That Is Not Protective for Osteoporosis

Weight-bearing activity has been studied, and is generally thought to be protective by increasing bone density. This will be discussed in detail in a separate section, along with its relevant research. As a logical extension, many researchers were not certain if obesity was protective for osteoporosis.

Using the data for male cadets can be helpful to examine this, as the military is well-funded to examine all of these aspects, and able to ensure high study compliance among its participants. In a lecture on femoral neck injuries, during basic training, Lt. Gen (ret.) Mark Hertling correlated an increased incidence of femoral neck fractures with obesity and climbing nutrition (see figure below).

Femoral Neck Injuries Encountered During Basic Training among new US Army Recruits at a Single Training Facility, 2000-2010

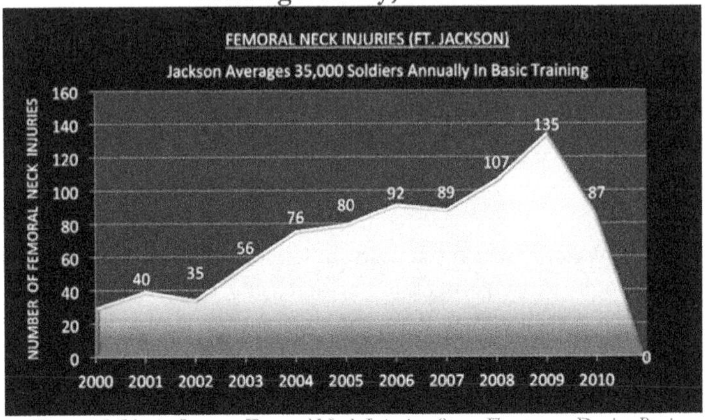

Figure 15 Obesity Impacts Femoral Neck Injuries -Stress Fractures - During Basic Training[139]

Indeed, the BMI of a new West Point (WP) or Citadel Military Academy Cadet has skyrocketed over time, as seen in the figure below:

BMI Values and Weight of an 18 year-old Cadet

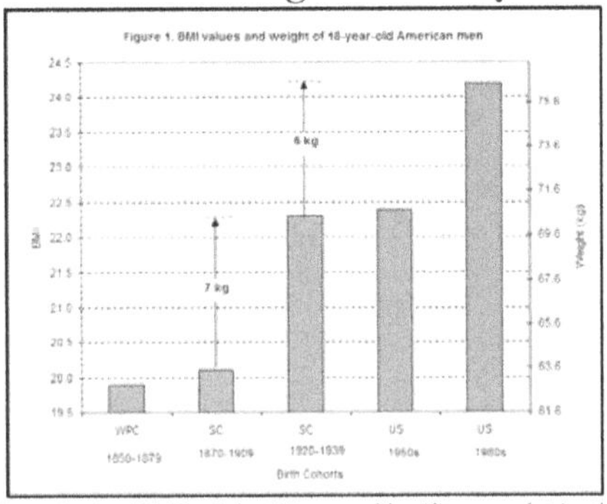

Figure 16 The skyrocketing BMI of the 18 year-old military cadet in the United States.

The chart also shows that the average weight of a 5 foot, 10 inch tall, 18 year-old has increased 15 kg approximately, from approximately 61 in 1850 to 76 kg in the 1980s.[140] Indeed, the population is getting larger, and yet obesity has not been shown to have any protective effect on reducing osteoporosis, when controlling for other risk factors.

Increased BMI is linked to Increased Bone Density, but Obesity is Not Protective for Osteoporosis

This is yet another example of how scientists are still learning about the basics of our bone physiology and architecture, and have a long way to go. Population studies, such as the Global Longitudinal Osteoporosis in Women Study (GLOW), shows that BMI may not directly correlate with overall fracture risk, but an increase in lower extremity fracture risk, while simultaneously resulting in fewer upper extremity fractures.[141] The challenge always lies in evaluating the numerous risk factors for osteoporosis.

Take for example, body-mass index, BMI, and it's role in osteoporosis. In one study, male volunteers aged 18-45 were screening for risk factors such as smoking, known endocrine disorders (eg. Diabetes) and medications that either directly or indirectly influence fat deposition. The screened 35 male participants underwent CT scanning to measure body fat and fat content of the bone marrow. What researchers found was an association between osteoporosis and fat deposition in the abdomen (visceral abdominal fat[8]), and an increased fat concentration in the bone marrow.[142] Then again, the authors observed that men with increase visceral abdominal fat and increased fat in the bone marrow among men with the same BMI had hormonal disorders, echoing the findings of other

[8] Visceral fat – within the peritoneal cavity/'abdominal' cavity, as compared with fat deposited in the layers underneath the skin, and above the abdominal layers.

studies as well.[143] Similarly, with muscle loss, in a study of psoas muscle size, decreased psoas muscle (psoas-muscle index) was associated with worsened bone density and increased fracture risk.[144]

Genetics of Bone Density

Numerous genes have been implicated in the process of bone development and bone pathology.[145] Having a family history of a compression fracture has been recognized as a significant risk factor and as a result has been included in the FRAX® 10-year risk assessment tool.

Some interesting genetic studies have been performed over the years to suggest a correlation between genetics and bone density. These genetic studies may compare monozygotic to dizygotic twins. Monozygotic twins are formed from one sperm and one egg, and are as a result, identical twins. Dizygotic twins result from two different sperm and two different eggs, each independent and each have unique genetics. Mikkola and coinvestigators then compared bone density parameters, finding a significantly higher intraclass correlation coefficient for bone characteristics within the Monozygotic (MZ) group (0.77-0.85 vs. 0.49-0.51 in dizygotic twins).[146] What this means is that the bone density findings were more consistent in the identical twin group pairs, suggesting a genetic component. While it is useful to see repeatable studies like these, it is important to be aware that monozygotic twins rely on foundational assumptions that monozygotic twins are genetically identical. Interestingly, this long held belief is being challenged.

Most people scratch their head at this statement and wonder why the author could dare say that identical twins are not at all identical. In modern times, long held dogma, when challenged, more dogma is created in response, all too often. In this case, the "environmental impacts" on the person's gene expression is used to explain unexpected findings of differing genetics. Here's where this get's interesting. In 2005, "Identical" (MZ) twins were compared in one study. Up to 35% of MZ twins differed later in life— a process called epigenetic effects. This was attributed to the environmental impact on the genes.[147] Subsequently, differences in the number of copies of a gene, called "copy number variants" were noted in a study of 19 sets of adult genetic twins ("identical twins").[148] This will be explained shortly. More recently, in *Nature Genetics*, Jonsson et al. found,

> "Here we show that monozygotic twins differ on average by 5.2 early developmental mutations and that approximately 15% of monozygotic twins have a substantial number of these early developmental mutations specific to one of them."[149]

So ultimately, over time, it is determined that from a "very early time" these twins have genetic differences. So then, how might one compare identical to fraternal twins in terms of risk factors? How much difference is acceptable?

From a practical standpoint, and for most patients, for most individual healthcare choices, genetics plays a limited role. The reason is due to a lack of understanding of the very basic mechanics of our DNA. Consider that our genome is 3 billion base pairs.[150] Of this massive library of base pairs, it was determined that between one and 2 percent of this DNA are used to create proteins that carry out essential processes of life, and the remainder are non-coding. Scientists had no understood function for 98-99% of our genome. Therefore, they called it junk DNA. In the mid-nineties, scientists were more openly discussing the many possible functions for "junk DNA".[151] Let's consider the 1972 article titled, "So much junk DNA" in our genome, and compare that to a special issue of *Molecular Genetics and Genomics* referred to by the editor as , "Junk DNA is not Junk."[152] In 2012, an online article titled, "What Junk DNA? It's an Operating System" writes:

> "Propelled by the publication of initial results in 2012 from the Encyclopedia of DNA Elements (ENCODE), a public research consortium launched by the U.S. National Human Genome Research Institute (NHGRI), scientists are increasingly identifying regulatory functions for intronic DNA. Publishing its initial findings in a set of 30 papers in Nature, Genome Biology, and Genome Research, ENCODE indicated that the biologically active portion of human DNA was "considerably higher" than any previous estimates. **In an overview paper, ENCODE reported that its members could assign biochemical functions to over 80% of the genome."**[153]

Ultimately, the point of the above digression was to convince the reader that the complex dynamics of the building blocks of life is so poorly understood, and it is not an understatement to say that the long-term impact of some established treatments may not be understood in entirety. One cannot be absolutely certain of all long-term impacts without fully understanding the mechanisms of the system (humans) that are being treated with medicines and other interventions.

Screening for Osteoporosis - Hip Fracture Risk

If anyone wants to know of one particular fracture that is devastating to the elderly, it is the "hip fracture", or the femoral neck. In particular, osteoporotic hip fractures occur primarily in elderly patients and in one study of patients who had a hip fractures, 30% of them died within one-year of the hip fracture. Although this could be for a number of reasons, it is for all of the things that can happen during the process of getting routine care for osteoporosis (the sequela).

Most often, it is due to the accumulating risk. Risk from numerous medical problems that develop in an elderly person who requires major surgery, general anesthesia, hospitalization, multiple injuries, infections, and the frequent other complications that occur along the way. Of the surviving 70% of patients in the aforementioned study, it is been observed that nearly half of those patients see a substantial decline in independence, and quality of life in general, with even 20% requiring nursing care on a long-term basis.[154]

Can Early Identification and Treatment of Osteoporosis result in a reduction in Fractures?

And here is where preventative measures such as screening and nutrition become most evident in terms of benefit— Early identification of osteoporosis and prompt treatment has been shown to result in a reduction in hip fractures. For women over 65, screening of osteoporosis and prompt treatment can provide a benefit in preventing fractures.

Primary Versus Secondary Osteoporosis

Osteoporosis, regardless of underlying cause, is still defined by the using bone densitometry (ie. DXA). Generally, one is said to have primary osteoporosis when it occurs in postmenopausal women. Primary osteoporosis in men occurs in the absence of an underlying cause. When a diagnosis of osteoporosis is attributed to an underlying cause, such as a disease or adverse effect of a medication, then that is referred to as secondary osteoporosis.[155] It is also associated with numerous diseases, chronic medication exposures, lifestyle, and the patient's risk for osteoporosis is often influenced by genetics.

Despite being so common, it never ceases to amaze the author when patients do not undergo screening, do not get a diagnostic workup, and available treatment, despite having a suspected osteoporotic fracture. Perhaps even more surprising are patients who get a diagnosis but do not follow-up and obtain the necessary treatment, which is often medication. This is clear evidence of a common perception that osteoporosis is less important that other chronic health conditions. It is understandable, because it is rarely a disease that prompts immediate preventative action.

Again, as far as healthcare professionals are concerned, the term primary osteoporosis refers to juvenile, postmenopausal, or osteoporosis in men and "senile" osteoporosis.[156] All other causes of osteoporosis attributed to various conditions and medications (Table below). Treatment and management of these are diagnosed by healthcare professionals and there diagnosis and workup process are extensive, often difficult. A discussion of these is beyond the scope of this book. Below are abbreviated Tables listing the numerous causes.

Secondary Osteoporosis – Related to Medication Use

Causes of Secondary Osteoporosis
Selective Serotonin Reuptake Inhibitors (SSRIs)
Proton Pump Inhibitors
Glucocorticoids
L-Thyroxin Suppressive Therapy
Heparin and Oral Anticoagulants
Thiazolidinediones
Anticonvulsants
Aromatase Inhibitors
Anti-retrovirals
Immunosuppressives
GnRH antagonists
Anti-androgens

Secondary Osteoporosis – Underlying conditions

Genetic (eg. Bone disorders)
Ehler-Danlos Syndrome
Osteogenesis Imperfecta
Marfan Syndrome
Cystic Fibrosis
Homocystinuria
Gaucher's Disease
Hypophosphatemia
Other Glycogen Storage Diseases
Rheumatoid arthritis
Ankylosing spondylitis
Psoriatic arthritis
Hyperparathyroidism
Diabetes mellitus
Hyperadrenocortisolism
Hypogonadism
Leukaemia
Multiple myeloma
Inflammatory bowel disease
Gastric surgery/gastrectomy/gastric bypass
COPD
Parkinson's
Multiple sclerosis

Secondary Osteoporosis- Lifestyle and Environmental Factors

Underweight (defined as BMI < 19 kg/m^2)
Insufficient Daily Calcium Intake (<1200 mg/day)
Smoking (most apparent when > 20 cigarettes/day)
Alcoholism (>60 g/day)[9]
Family History of osteoporosis

---

[9] In the United States, there is 14 grams of alcohol in a can (12 oz, or 355 mL) of beer, 5 ounces of win (150 mL), or 1.5 ounces of liquor ("spirit"). 157 Nuti, R., Brandi, M., G, C. & al., e. Guidelines for the management of osteoporosis and fragility fractures. **14**, 86-88 (2019). If the alert reader then asks, how can just over 4 cans of beer be defined as alcoholism? The National Institute on Alcohol Abuse and Alcoholism (NIAAA), a branch of the larger National Institute of Health (NIH), defines heavy alcohol use as: "For men, consuming more than 4 drinks on any day or more than 14 drinks per week." And "For women, consuming more than 3 drinks on any day or more than 7 drinks per week."

7 Diagnosis

One of the difficulties with raising public awareness of osteoporosis, is due to the clinically silent course throughout the development of decreased bone density. It presents itself as a problem only after a fracture occurs. In many instances, even in patients with a new fracture following a trauma, such as a motor vehicle collision, many patients do not see the importance, because they have a readily explainable cause of the fracture— ie., the motor vehicle did it, and it was expected.

In a survey of 430 women, approximately half had knowledge of osteoporosis, and about half of all participants had a positive attitude about preventative care. Despite knowledge and positive attitude, the study revealed a degree of ambivalance, in that, by and large, they did not indicate that they were taking preventative measures.[158]

How Is Osteoporosis Diagnosed?

Treating the problem begins with *identifying the problem.* In modern medicine, consistent diagnostic methods are important for ensuring that patients receive treatment in line with recommendations or guidelines. Standardization of care is an important issue but for the process of osteoporosis this digression can be avoided.

Can Compression Fractures be Diagnosed by Physical Examination, *without Imaging*?

The physical examination performed by a physician will not produce any findings that are unique to compression fractures alone. Sure, with an appropriate history and physical examination, it could be reliably suspected, but confirmation will require advanced imaging. Also, a combination of a mild injury mechanism and severe back pain may suggest an osteoporotic compression fracture, but this diagnosis likewise cannot be made with any degree of certainty without medical imaging. Commonly, the only findings of compression fractures are spine tenderness, and with enough severity, a change in the normal spine contour can be felt (palpated), indicating kyphosis.[159]

A diagnosis of osteoporosis relies heavily on bone densitometry, measured by a dual-energy x-ray absorptiometry (DEXA) method. This method of measuring the density of the bones utilizes a specialized type of x-ray machine, apart from the x-ray machine used to detect fractures (see figure below).

Bone Densitometry

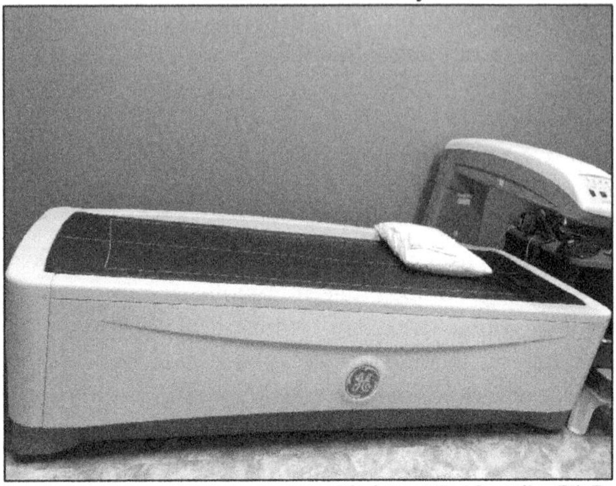

Figure 17. Bone Densitometry Scanning Machine; GE, Norwalk, CT. Reprinted from The Neck Pain Guide (Ghobrial, 2020).

Bone density is measured by the DEXA method, and compared to a reference table of averages. So, the standard deviation (SD) above or below the mean peak bone mass (Fig.), is also called the T-Score. The T-score is not just a comparison of the mean, but it is a comparison to the average bone mass in a thirty year-old, healthy adult. Therefore, osteoporosis is defined as more than 2.5 SD below the mean, which is the same as saying '< -2.5 SD' in a report. When the threshold is between -2.5 and -1, this is called 'osteopenia', which is the same as saying that one has decreased bone density and may be at risk. And so, the 'normal' bone density in medicine is referred to as a score between -1 to +2.5 SD.

Bone Densitometry and Reliability Issues in the Lumbar Spine

Many authors have written that BMD does not predict spinal fracture risk, advocating for other methodology to evaluate the spine.[160] After all, with advances in technology and our ability to resolve the finer three dimensional structure of bone, perhaps with further research a more predictive tool can be created. Specifically singling out dual-energy x-ray absorptiometry, it's assessment of the lumbar spine may be less reliable simply due to even minor technique differences among x-ray technicians, such as positioning, machine calibration, institutional protocols, and technician experience-level. All are likely to contribute to significant variance in results.[43] To further stress this importance, in "DXA Quality Matters", Lewiecki opines:

> "Contrary to the common misperception that BMD measurement and interpretation is a simple procedure requiring no special expertise, densitometer maintenance/operation, data acquisition, and interpretation/reporting of the results are skills that must be acquired and maintained. We recommend that technologists and clinicians involved with performing or interpreting BMD tests be educated and trained in bone densitometry and that they update their skills regularly. We also suggest that they provide demonstration of proficiency in bone densitometry in order to assure patients, referring healthcare providers, and payers of medical services that these skills have been acquired and maintained."[161]

Assessing the hypothesis that DXA does not provide a reliable assessment of "bone quality" of the lumbar spine, Pumberger and coinvestigators performed biopsies of patients with and without lumbar fractures, comparing bone densitometry to micro-CT. They assessed for a correlation between DXA results, micro-CT findings, and the architecture of the bone obtained from the biopsy, and in general attempted to correlate quality with the presence of lumbar spinal fractures.[162] "Micro-CT" is a type of CT test that provides tissue characterization.[163] What they found was that while micro-CT findings correlated with worsening bone quality, lumbar bone densitometry "...neither qualitatively nor quantitatively represented microstructural bone architecture and was therefore not a reliable tool for the evaluation of bone quality in the spine."

In a prior study, the authors assessed an alternate candidate to DXA for assessing bone quality of the lumbar spine, the high-resolution multidetector CT.[164] However, they did not find this device to be a successful candidate as a screening tool, having a poor correlation. Indeed, it will be some time before a suitable tool is designed, identified, and introduced into use.

WHO Grading of Osteoporosis

Meanwhile, bone densitometry is the standard for grading bone mineral density and diagnosing osteoporosis. The World Health Organization (WHO) defines osteoporosis in relative terms of BMD. The values of BMD are not as one would expect as a density measurement, ie., mass over volume, grams per millimeter cubed, one would expect with density. Instead, relative values of bone density are used and there are always a smaller percentage of individuals with bone density well below the mean.

For standardization of treatment, the WHO recommends bone density to be graded using the following guidelines[165]:

1. Normal: +2.5 to -1 SD
2. Osteopenia (low bone density): -1 to -2.5 SD
3. Osteoporosis: less than -2.5 SD
4. Severe Osteoporosis: less than -2.5 *and* one or more fragility fracture.

To explain this matter further, bone density, and other attributes of a large adult population is expected to follow a Gaussian Distribution, which to most people is commonly known as the Bell Curve (except at the Gauss Family Dinner Table). A Bell Curve fits certain characteristics, such as having only one peak, where most values, for example, T-scores, are distributed near the average (see figure below).

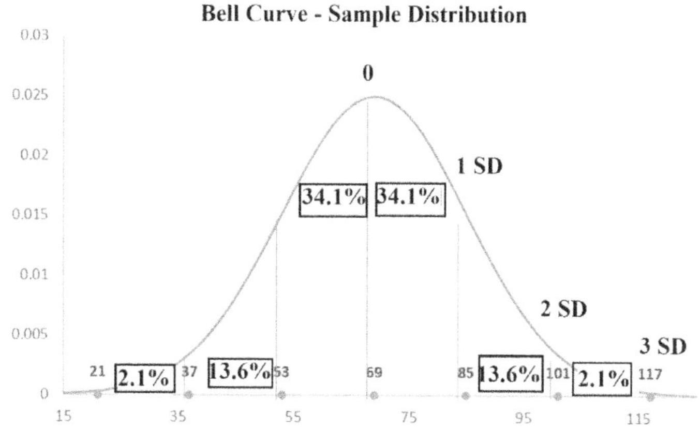

Figure 18. The Bell Curve, or Gaussian Distribution, with percentiles of corresponding standard deviations. The y- axis is the defined distribution, such as bone densitometry measurement, and the x-axis is expressed as a measure representing the frequency of the value, standard deviation, or percent. For example, 1 standard deviations above and below the mean represents approximately 68.2%, 2 deviations represents approximately 95% of the population.

In general, decreased bone mineral density (BMD) is a major risk for fracture. Numerous other risk factors predispose one to fragility fractures: among these less clearly defined factors include bone structural factors ('the bone architecture'), as well as age, a previous history of fragility fractures, corticosteroid use, other secondary and genetic causes of osteoporosis, and even conditions that can predispose a patient to falls.

If There Are So Many Risk Factors for Fracture, How is Bone Densitometery the Most Important?

There are many reasons why bone densitometry is chiefly used to diagnosis osteoporosis, but at the present time, it is practical, and it correlates well with preventing hip fractures, which have the most devastating impact. There are many risk factors, but none of which can be standardized and measured across all patients. Additionally, scientific research studies show a relationship between worsening BMD and increased fractures. In general, for every decrease (loss) in bone density by 1 SD, the risk of fracture increases by a factor of 1.5-3.[166]

A CT Scan Is Not Yet An Acceptable Substitute For A DEXA Scan

Patients routinely undergo computed tomography (CT) scanning in the process to diagnosis potential fractures and characterize them for treatment purposes. These fractures commonly include areas such as the lumbar spine and hip-region that are routinely scanned during bone densitometry for the routine screening for osteoporosis. Also, the same test is used to diagnose a spine or femoral neck fracture, and the question comes as to whether a CT can replace the DEXA study (bone densitometry), both as a matter of saving money, saving time, and getting additional use out of a wealth of information that most likely contains the information needed to determine bone density. This is all, just a matter of time, with regards to a CT being used to determine BMD. As mentioned earlier, there are still limitations of the current tools at determining biomechanical characteristics of bone.

In some instance, patients may be told that they “may”, or “possibly” have osteoporosis, based off of a CT. What is the basis for making this statement, if any? Well, again, this is just an appearance on CT scan, and that further workup is advised, even without evidence of a fracture. Is there an underlying basis for this recommendation, if any? Well, these guidelines are based off of extensive clinical experience and a growing body of research studies. Formally, CT scans are not a standard method for diagnosis and treatment. Also, a CT scan, depending on the specific test, ranges from significantly more, to vastly more radiation than bone densitometry.

On CT scan, density is approximated by measuring Hounsfeld Units, a measure of brightness on CT, or the appreciation of decreased signal on a plain film (x-ray).[10] While the "brightness" of a CT or X-ray, is often due to numerous fractures, including technique, body weight, and other factors such as the thickness of tissue over the specific bone of interest. Observe the CT scan of the lumbar spine below, obtained in a 70 year-old woman with back pain after a fall from standing (figure 19 below). She has not had a workup for osteoporosis before. While there appears to be a significant decrease in the visualized bone, this is not diagnostic for osteoporosis as the definitions are based off of T-scores obtained from bone densitometry.

Compression Fractures

As mentioned above, one of the main jobs of the spine is to serve as a column to allow for us to walk upright, and to serve as a load-bearing column. Failure of that column can occur with osteoporosis, where the vertebral body undergoes a compression fracture. These fractures affecting the vertebral body, causing them to become shorter. There are numerous classifications of compression fractures and naming schemes that were designed by physicians for the use by healthcare providers to facilitate decision making and research. These systems of classification are closely linked to surgical management, radiology, intensive critical, and other disciplines— with this book being a discussion of osteoporosis and management of the most common problems, a detailed discussion of compression fractures will not include other axial compression mechanisms such as "burst" fractures, fracture

---

[10] The Hounsfeld Units is also referred to as a "CT Unit" less commonly, and is a relative measurement of "radio density". The density of different bodily tissues are related to a grayscale of brightness, with the brightest values meant to represent the highest densities. An excellent explanation is provided by the NCBI at https://www.ncbi.nlm.nih.gov/books/NBK547721/.

classification systems, spinal stabilization surgery, and other complex emergencies.

Compression fractures can occur from what patients may describe as nontraumatic, even trivial events, or no clearly recognizable event at all. In some instances, patients with coughing, sneezing, or twisting can precipitate a compression fracture.

Lumbar Spine CT Scan Demonstrating a Mild Osteoporotic Compression Fracture

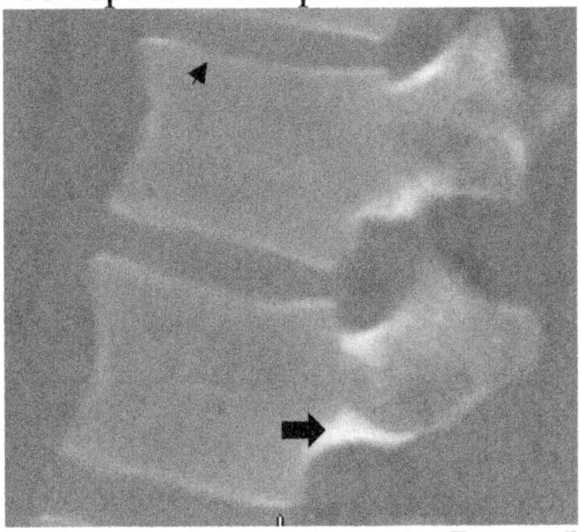

Figure 19 Mild Age-indeterminate Compression Fracture, CT scan, sagittal projection. On a CT scan, this fracture occurs in the superior endplate (small arrow). Note the relatively brighter appearance (broad arrow) seen which corresponds with increased density ie. less radiation can penetrate through and be detected).

Note in the aforementioned figure, a thin, faint rim of cortical bone is observed through the endplate. A general decrease in the apparent density of the bone can be appreciated in the vertebral body, but the density cannot be measured by CT. CT is currently not considered a criterion for a diagnosis of osteoporosis. Observe the next CT of the thoracic spine below, and appreciate this relatively more advanced loss in bone mineralization (see figure 20 below).

Thoracic Spine CT Scan In an Elderly Trauma Patient with Osteoporosis

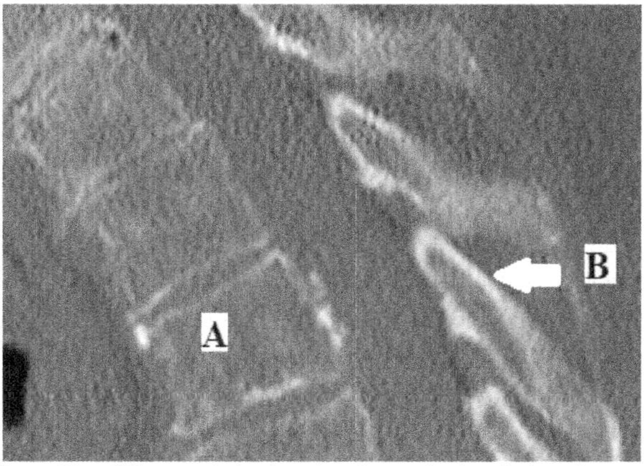

Figure 20. CT scan of the thoracic spine, sagittal projection, demonstrating a magnified view of the vertebral bodies of the thoracic spine, with a suspected vertebral body (A). Compared to the previous figure, one can appreciate the significant differences in the lack of signal in the spine. Posteriorly, one can also appreciate the increased signal in the posterior laminar bone (B) which is very bright and several millimeters in thickness and it is common to be able to see relatively large differences in apparent bone mineralization across the spinal structures in the same person.

While a CT scan is not used to provide a formal diagnosis of osteoporosis, much research has been conducted in the past 10 years to help physicians frame a narrative with a patient who has no prior screening and a recent CT scan. In the case of a spine fracture in a trauma patient, very often that person who sustains a fracture will be told that they likely have osteoporosis based off of a CT, which is common. Most often they are correct. The CT scan and discussion often occurs in the emergency department (ED) or urgent care center for an injury.

The overall goal of these endeavors is to improve efficiency, prevent or reduce complications, promote wellness for patients, and at the same time this reduces costs and hopefully improve quality of life. The emergency department is not the only time that a patient will undergo a CT. Therefore, there are potentially many areas that a patient may have the opportunity to have their bone evaluated, should a validated algorithm be identified one day that can diagnose osteoporosis. In one study, patient's underwent HU measurement in the leg, obtained during the process of a screening test, a CT colonoscopy.[11] The USPSTF provides guidance on colorectal cancer screening guidelines, usually with a colonscopy[133], which is a separate procedure called a CT colonoscopy. Indications for the CT colonscopy are beyond the scope of this discussion. Nonetheless, this gastrointestinal study aims to determine if CT scanning that normally includes views of the proximal femur in the periphery, the same location scanned during a DEXA study, could provide equally useful information for the workup of osteoporosis. The researchers in this study closely approximated the location where a DEXA scan would be obtained to provide a consistent measure of HU, that could serve as a surrogate marker. Ultimately, the researchers found that the measure of the femur during the CT colonscopy had a high correlation (0.75) to DEXA scans.[133] In other words, as reported in this study, CT colonoscopy demonstrated promise as a test where bone density may in the future be measured.

Hounsfield Units and The CT Scan

The Hounsfield Unit is a measurement of density on a CT scan, expressed in terms of Hounsfield Units (HU) and most often ranges from -1000 for air, to +1000 for dense bone, and even nearly to 2000 in cranial bone. There are extended ranges where these measurements go higher, but air is calibrated to -1000 and distilled water is calibrated to zero. So, what would be the measurement of foreign bodies? In one report, the maximum upper limit is 30,000 for gold, steel, and brass.[167]

---

[11] The US. Preventative Services Task Force recommends that all adults aged 50-75 be screened for colorectal cancer. For ages 50-75, they provide a "Grade A" recommendation, which is the highest grade of recommendation, viz. "There is a high certainty that the net benefit is substantial." Grades B and C are for decreasing certainty and potential benefit, Grade D is a recommendation against a treatment (Grade D - discourage), and Grade I is given whenever inadequate information is available.

Therefore, in one review of the literature, general parameters were suggested that would correlate HU to bone density:

Correlating CT to Bone Density, Results From a Systematic Review[16]

HU Range	Classification of Bone Density
54.7-130	Osteoporotic Bone
78.8-146	Osteopenic
120.8-230	Normal

Researchers have found CT measures of HU of kidney stones to be helpful to the point of recommending HU considerations in the management of kidney stones, due to the potential nonresponse of certain treatments to relatively higher HU stones.[168] Conflicting evidence does exist as to the accuracy and relationship between measurement of HU and Bone Density and this is mainly because HU is semi-quantitative, and only an approximation, applied to a linear scale whereby air is assigned the value of value, arbitrarily.

Lumbar Spine Hounsfield Unit Measurement and Bone Density

The lumbar spine is of specific interest to the reader. How helpful are HU with regards to the lumbar and thoracolumbar spine? The majority of lumbar fractures occur at the thoracolumbar junction, including the first and second lumbar segments. There have been a number of studies in the last ten years that look at the lumbar spine specifically in terms of HU measurements and bone density. Again, conflicting results are obtained across the many studies, but it appears that over time, with the development of the importance of consistency, accuracy, and a precise form of measurement, there may be promise for using a lumbar CT to one day replace the DEXA scan and provide both a fracture screening and bone density measurement simultaneously. Therefore, if the test does not show a fracture, data on bone density will substantially shorten the wait time for a patient to receive treatment.

As a reminder, first and foremost, regardless of how valuable this research is, osteopenia and osteoporosis are standardized definitions of the World Health Organization and therefore the only time a CT scan will substitute for a DEXA scan is in the future after societies change their guidelines. Nonetheless, varying results are obtained across lumbar spine studies, and two meta-analyses are worth mentioning. In 2019, a meta-analysis[12] of 9 studies published in the journal *Spine* compared CT measurements of HU to bone densitometry of the lumbar spine, and found no clear correlation between the two.[169] In other words, they did not find this avenue to be fruitful across the results of 9 studies. And yet, only 2 years later, in 2021, a meta-analysis of 18 studies was published in the same journal, enrolling far more patients, 5307, comparing T-scores and HU measurements of the lumbar spine, and found "favorable results" for correlating the lumbar spine T-score with the HU measurement.[170] Again, across numerous studies, the value of measuring HU and using it as a diagnostic tool will be some time before enough research is completed to allow healthcare leaders to formalize different recommendations, whenever they are indicated as a potential future substitutes for the DEXA study.

Measuring Lumbar HU as a Predictive Tool for Compression Fracture Risk

Previously, it was asked if HU could be a surrogate tests for the DEXA test. However, has it been shown if HU values correspond to fracture risk, independent to the DEXA study? Perhaps this would simplify the process, by showing a direct correlate to a clinical outcome, allow for researchers to

---

[12] A meta-analysis attempts to quantify the data from multiple similar studies, whenever possible, in an attempt to gain greater insight from multiple, small, often conflicting studies. The pros and cons of this study, especially the potential errors of these types of "studies" should be understood and an excellent paper by Eysenck, titled, "Meta-analysis and its problems" can be found on the National Library of Medicine Website (https://pubmed.ncbi.nlm.nih.gov/7950571/)

overcome the hurdle of showing a correlation between two tests. One of the problems with this is in realizing that the lumbar spine is a load-bearing structure and perhaps some vertebral bodies require a greater integrity than others, due to their weight, or other spinal biomechanics such as global spinal alignment.

Regardless, patients diagnosed with fractures were compared to controls, in a study of almost 2000 patients looking at HU measures. Graffy and coinvestigators measured the L1 vertebral body, and the resulting HU from CT scan in 1966 consecutive patients, finding a mean L1 HU measurement of 70.2 among those with a spine fracture and a HU of 132.3 in participants without a spine fracture. The likelihood of a moderate or severe compression fracture increased from 32.5 to 49.2% when the HU measurement decreased from ≤ 90 to ≤50.[171] As we see here, this substantial difference, if repeatable in larger studies, may be an alternate avenue to develop the HU as a test.

In determining fracture risk, researchers have been looking at whether CTs of the abdomen obtained in the emergency department, for instance, could provide an excellent opportunity to measure the density (by HU) of the lumbar spine and provide a measure of fracture risk.[169] Outside of the emergency department, similar feasibility has been assessed in the setting of an oncology practice, where CTs are frequently obtained to assess cancer status.[172]

In a hypothetical example, suppose a patient was undergoing workup for severe abdominal pain and eventually, a CT was ordered of the abdomen, after treatment of the abdominal pain, the patient would be notified that a low density scan is predictive of elevated fracture risk. They would then be given a referral for medical workup for osteoporosis. Since the abdominal CT is limited to the abdomen, researchers have looked at Chest CT studies as well and have found that they are similarly helpful in assessing bone density of the thoracic spine.[173] In one study of 140 patients with planned spinal surgery, HU was found to be a more accurate prognostication tool than bone densitometry (ie. T-scores) for determining if a patient would have an osteoporosis-related postoperative complication.[174] In another related study, Lee and coinvestigators identified 204 patients who sustained a hip fracture, and underwent CT of the abdomen just prior to treatment . The goal was to identify risk factors for hip fracture. In order to do so, they compared these patients with age and gender-matched controls, that is to say, similar patients in general risk, but without a hip fracture. What they found was that a decrease in HU of the trabecular bone of either the L1 spinal vertebral body or the femoral neck[13], and/or the presence of at least one spinal compression fracture was predictive of a hip fracture.[175]

Osteoporosis Predicts Complications Following Spinal Surgery and Other Orthopedic Surgeries

There is also evidence that low bone density inferred by Hus from CT, or by DEXA can complicate surgical outcomes, particular those that require implants such as screws, pins, and other implants that interface metallic implants, "cement" polymers, with a bone surface. In one study, patients with osteopenia (T-scores less than one), were associated with a higher likelihood of an osteoporosis-related complication (ORCs). The overall incidence of ORCs was close to one-third of all patients in this study.[176]

Often, depending on the goals of spinal surgery involved an instrumented fusion, which is the mobilization of a single motion segment in the spine, using screws, rods, and occasionally other implants, such as cages to maintain or restore anatomic alignment and motion.

Most importantly, this avenue of research would be very beneficial to the patient and society in general, limiting

---

[13] Trabecular bone is the majority of the volume of the vertebral body, and it is surrounded by a denser superficial layer of cortical bone, an arrangement found throughout the skeleton.

additional tests, lowering costs, and shortening wait times. Moreover, any attempts to lower radiation exposure to the patient will lower the number of radiation-induced tumors, some of which can be life- threatening malignancies.

The United States Preventive service task force screening: Recommendations for Osteoporosis

Before entering a discussion of recommendations, it is important to understand how many scientists grade medical evidence. As the author has mentioned in *The Low Back Pain Guide* and *The Neck Pain Guide*, not all areas of medicine are studied intensely for a myriad of reasons. Excellent studies are very expensive, time-consuming, and since funding is finite, common diseases (high prevalence) will be expected to have more research studies and of greater quality.

The United States Preventive Services Task Force (USPSTF) is an independent panel of experts that make evidence-based recommendations specifically for public health issues and as the says it, are focused on disease prevention. Things that one will find are 'guidelines' for screening and preventative treatments. Since inception in 1984, the USPSTF has grown in size and in relevance in US healthcare. In recognition of that, The Agency for Healthcare Research and Quality (AHRQ), a division of the US Department of Health and Human Services, began funding, administrating, and directing the mission of the USPSTF, which, arguably exerts majority if not complete management of this "independent" agency after 1998.

The USPSTF uses a grading scale as shown below, in order to provide further recommendations for the screened patient. Again, as mentioned above, not all recommendations can be made with the same quality of research. As expected, grade A is the highest recommendation and implies a substantial benefit can be expected when a recommendation is adhered to by the provider. This is followed by grade B, C, and D, for discouraging the use of a particular treatment or service. Instead of F, grade I means that there is insufficient evidence for, or against a recommendation and there is uncertainty about benefit or harm from a treatment or recommendation (see table below, adapted from USPSTF).[177]

USPSTS Grades of Recommendation

Grade	Definition	Suggestions For Practice
A	The USPSTF recommends the service. Highly likely to be beneficial.	Recommend/ Provide
B	The USPSTF recommends the service. There is at least moderate likelihood that the net benefit is moderate or greater.	Recommend/ Provide
C	The USPSTF recommends treatment for specific populations, or "Case-by-Case" basis.	Recommend/Provide when individual criteria met.
D	The USPSTF recommends against implementing a measure/treatment/service.	Do not recommend.
I	Evidence is insufficient, poor, or conflicting.	In general, do not recommend.

Evidence exists in support of the practice of osteoporosis screening as early detection can help prevent fractures so long as early detection is followed by treatment. Treatment is usually in the form of medication to decrease processes that break down bone and with some medications facilitate bone growth or mineralization. The USPSTF recommends screening for women 65 years and older. For women at risk under the age of 65, early detection of osteoporosis is also thought to be beneficial (See table below).[178]

USPSTF Summary Recommendations for Osteoporosis Prevention

Population	Recommendation	Great
Women ≥65 years	USPSTF recommends osteoporosis screening with 'bone measurement testing.'	B
Women <65 years, postmenopausal or at increased risk	USPSTF recommends osteoporosis screening with 'bone measurement testing.	B
Men	Insufficient evidence.	I

Bone measurement testing typically refers to dual X-ray absorptiometry (DEXA) which provides an assessment of bone mineral density (BMD) which is known to correlate with one's risk of fracture, when left untreated. As mentioned above, this is recommended by the WHO.

Osteoporotic Compression Fractures: CT Imaging and Bone Density is a New Area Highlighted Research

Compression fractures are very common, and this is most often due to osteoporosis and mild trauma. Compression fractures themselves are typically diagnosed by CT. Pickhardt and colleagues as well as others have noted for some time that CT imaging, with greater research, may become excellent surrogate studies for the assessment of bone density as well.[179] Please see the preceding section regarding the extensive research in this area.

8 Risk Factors

Risk factors for the development of Osteoporosis are numerous and most often multifactorial. While genetics has a major role in the physiology of bone mineralization and turnover, the majority of osteoporosis causes are lifestyle- related. Medications that pose a known risk factor to osteoporosis will be discussed. These are commonly used in the treatment of chronic medical conditions such as hypertension and diabetes, elevating their importance in the identification as potential risk factors.

Medications That Potentially Increase Risk for Osteoporosis

A myriad of medications are *associated* with decreased bone density, and the development of osteopenia and osteoporosis. The educated reader should not burden themselves with memorizing the contents of these lists, nor should they be tasked with carrying the authors various handbooks with them to each appointment. Benjamin Franklin once said, "an ounce of prevention is worth a pound of cure", albeit he stated this in regards to funding a fire department *before* the fire.

The long-term use of specific medications to treat chronic diseases is occasionally linked to drugs that may very well be associated with the loss of BMD. Below is a table listing just a some of the common medications that are associated with the development of osteoporosis (see table below).

Medications associated with the development of osteoporosis[180]

Glucocorticoids
Proton pump inhibitors
Selective serotonin re-uptake inhibitors
Anticonvulsants
L-thyroxine suppressive therapy
Aromatase inhibitors
Immunosuppressives
GnRH antagonists
Heparin
Oral anticoagulants
Thiazolidinediones

Corticosteroids and The Risk of Osteoporosis

Since that is a very broad list, one or two relatively more common medications should be discussed, due to their widespread use. Corticosteroids are a general class of medication, and act as an immunosuppressant, or a potent anti-inflammatory medication. Chronic corticosteroid use is estimated to occur in up to 1% of the US population, in the form of glucocorticoids.[181] Why so many? Most often, this is due to long term treatment of chronic obstructive pulmonary disease (COPD) with corticosteroids. Examples of glucocorticoids include cortisone, hydrocortisone, and prednisone (see table below).

Abbreviated List of Common Glucocorticoids

Glucocorticoid	Potency	Relative Duration of Effect	Mineralocorticoid Potency
Cortisone/Cortisol	0.9	Short	0.9
Hydrocortisone-Hydrocortisol	1.0	Short	1.0
Prednisone/Prednisolone	4.0	Intermediate	0.6
Methylprednisolone	5.0	Intermediate	0.6
Triamcinolone	5.0	Intermediate	0
Fludrocortisone	10	Long	125
Dexamethasone	30.0	Long	0
Betamethasone	35.0	Long	0

Table 3 List of common glucocorticoids and their relative potencies. Relative potencies in this table closely approximate hydrocortisone equivalency but are not reliable in this fashion, as several medications are topical formulations only (ie. skin creams). Also shown are the relative duration of effect, and mineralocorticoid potency.

Evidence from clinical trials and further medical literature suggests a relationship between increased daily dosage of glucocorticoids and increased fracture risk.[182-186] It is observed that most bone loss occurs not in the first 3 months, but after 3 to 6 months of glucocorticoid use.[187] There is a lack of research supporting any association between short-term steroid use for acute low back and leg pain and any influence on the development of osteoporosis. This is most likely because it is the daily exposure of corticosteroids. Corticosteroids upset the balance of bone turnover by preventing new bone formation altogether while stimulating the formation of osteoclasts, cells that only break down bone.[188] One study by Van Staa et al., found that at doses of 30 mg or greater, or beyond a total daily dose of five grams, there was a greater risk for hip and spinal fractures.[189]

9 The Medical Management of Osteoporosis

The strategy for managing osteoporosis is tailored to the patient, as well as the goals of care. The treatment of osteoporotic compression fractures is different and addressed in the sections later in this book. Overall, most patients fit into the following four groups, each of which require a unique strategy.

1. Screening for osteoporosis/osteopenia
2. Correction of osteoporosis/osteopenia
3. Osteoporotic Fragility Fracture Care
4. Prevention of Subsequent Fragility Fractures

Medications For the Prevention or Management of Osteoporosis

For better or worse, medications serve as the mainstay of treatment of osteoporosis. In general, treating osteoporosis means to improve bone density or prevent the worsening of BMD. This in turn will help lower the risk of a compression fracture, or subsequent osteoporotic fracture elsewhere, such as in one's arms or legs, which was discussed in detail above. For example, lifestyle modification and diet are arguably important factors as well. Focusing on prescription medications at this time, numerous drugs are approved for the prevention of osteoporotic fractures. These are most generally classified into two groups: anti-resorptive agents and anabolic agents. One note for the interested reader. These lists are constantly in a state of flux, due to new guidelines and every so often, a new warning, or the introduction of new medications and alterations to dosing. So, this is meant to serve as a brief primer. Due to the number of options, one may ask themselves how does one choose from so many options? Well, in this case, a healthcare expert will be the prescriber of these medications. And, that person would gladly explain how a particular recommendation was arrived at. Treatments are tailored to an individual.

Antiresorptives

These include estrogen, calcitonin, bisphosphonates, raloxifene, and denosumab. These inhibit osteoclasts activity which results in less bone resorption. This results in increased bony mineralization. Mineralization is what is measured on bone mineral density testing.

Denosumab

Of these listed, denosumab is the newest antiresorptive, approved in 2010. As a monoclonal antibody to RANKL, the end result of binding this receptor results in significant increases in BMD.[190] Denosumab is somewhat different than the bisphosphonates, in that it undergoes less of a plateau in BMD increase with continued use. However, when discontinuing Denosumab, there is a greater risk for rebound loss in BMD, and another bisphosphonate agent may be part of the planned therapy to prevent rapid bone loss from occurring.

Anabolic agents

Anabolic agents differ from above, in that they directly stimulate bone growth.[188] Three anabolic agents are approved for use in osteoporosis, with some caveats. Due to the potential adverse events associated with these medications, knowledge of these risks is vital to informed consent. Some patients have higher risks for these potentially fatal complications and therefore the determination of which patients are appropriate for these medications is made by the patient as well as their prescribing physician.

Strontium Ranelate

Strontium ranelate is not FDA approved in the United States. It is however, worthy of discussion to illustrate the potential risks of medications and why it is important to discuss these medications with a physician. They are not to be taken lightly. Strontium ranelate was approved in Australia and in the UK for the treatment of osteoporosis. It was marked for its unique "dual-action" in that it both increased osteoblast activity, and decreases osteoclast activity, both of which lead to a potent effect in bone turnover that favors the deposition of bone.[191] Strontium ranelate is of interest due to evidence showing that it may reduce the risk of both spinal and non-spinal fractures.[192] One avenue of research is currently under preclinical investigation is the coating of spinal interbody implants, such as PEEK cages with strontium ranelate to accelerate bone growth during a spinal fusion.[193]

So what are the risks of Strontium ranelate? Strontium is a trace metal, nearly all of which is concentrated in the bones. Due to similarities to calcium, strontium can displace calcium and potential lead to a falsely elevate BMD. Also, serious life threatening risks have been reported. Said *American Bone Health* in their bulletin:

> "Taking strontium supplements for any period of time is likely to make future bone density tests inaccurate. (Strontium may remain in the bones for as long as 7–10 years after the last dose.) … Because strontium atoms are heavier than calcium atoms, swapping some of the calcium atoms with strontium atoms will make the bone mineral density appear to increase. This is not the same as making new bone…**Research from Europe suggests that patients on**

> **strontium ranelate may have an increased risk of heart attacks, blood clots, and serious skin reactions (DRESS syndrome).”** [192]

Teriparatide

Teriparatide, an anabolic agent, is the first bone anabolic agent in use in the United States. This drug is injected subcutaneously on a daily basis, for up to two years. This drug has a similar molecular appearance to human parathyroid hormone, allowing it to act as a synthetic hormone (hence, it is an anabolic agent). The net result is the increase in bone density via the conversion of stem cells into osteoblasts and other supportive cells that increase in bone formation.[194] It is important to keep in mind that teriparatide (trade name: Forteo®) is FDA-approved for preventative indications, however the FDA approval letter states:

> “FORTEO is indicated for the treatment of postmenopausal women with osteoporosis who are at high risk for fracture. These include women with a history of osteoporotic fracture, or who have multiple risk factors for fracture, or who have failed or are intolerant of previous osteoporosis therapy, based upon physician assessment (*see* BLACK BOX WARNING). In postmenopausal women with osteoporosis, FORTEO increases BMD and reduces the risk of vertebral and nonvertebral fractures. FORTEO is indicated to increase bone mass in men with primary or hypogonadal osteoporosis who are at high risk for fracture. These include men with a history of osteoporotic fracture, or who have multiple risk factors for fracture, or who have failed or are intolerant to previous osteoporosis therapy, based upon physician assessment (*see* BLACK BOX WARNING). In men with primary or hypogonadal osteoporosis, FORTEO increases BMD. The effects of FORTEO on risk for fracture in men have not been studied.”[195]

The FDA uses the term "black-box warning" to call attention to very serious or potentially life-threatening risks. For FORTEO™, that is the potential risk of osteosarcoma, a malignant bone cancer with a high mortality rate. This risk was derived from experimental rat studies, where rats were followed at 6, 20, and 24 months at doses of 0, 5, and 30 mcg/day. They found a significantly higher incidence of bone cancers in the higher dose group. Registries have been established to monitor for the occurrence of cancer, and the black-box warning has been placed until these matters are researched in further detail.[196]

Most importantly, it is important to understand that these osteoporosis medications, including Forteo™ are approved for the treatment of osteoporosis, but the guidelines outside of that, such as for the treatment of fractures, are different. The North American Menopause Society, in a 2006 Guideline proposed that Teriparatide by reserved for only those at relatively greater risk for osteoporotic fractures—specifically it was proposed for women with a T-score less than 3.0.[197]

Abaloparatide

Abaloparatide is another parathyroid-like molecule/protein that has a similar effect of teriparatide. The potency may be less, however.

Romosozumab

A third agent is Romosozumab; this is a monoclonal antibody which is a molecule made in a laboratory structured in a manner similar to an antibody in the natural immune system, designed to bind and inhibits sclerostin. Sclerostin and is a molecule that by itself, inhibits bone formation. So the inhibitor of an inhibitor results in the overall increase in bone formation. In fact, there are dramatic results.

Ibandronate

Ibandronate is a relatively newer bisphosphonate, among the most potent bisphosphonates.

Abbreviated Selection of Medications for the Preventation of Osteoporosis, as Reported by the American Association of Family Practitioners

Medication	Dosage (mg)	Frequency	Mechanism
Alendronate	5	Daily	Antiresorptive
Ibandronate	150	Monthly	Antiresorptive
Risendronate	5	Daily*	Antiresorptive
Zoledronic Acid	5	Single dose, every other year	Antiresorptive
Calcium	1,000-1,200	Daily	Antiresorptive
Estrogen	0.3-0.625	Daily	Antiresorptive

*Table 4 Medications for the Treatment of Osteoporosis, as Reported by the AAFP in 2016. Adapted from "Diagnosis and Management of Vertebral Compression Fractures"[198] Medications described above are for personal educational only, which may raise one's informed consent when they make a decision with their trusted healthcare provider. Trade names are omitted. *-monthly frequency available.*

Brief Summary

In summary, there are number of therapies available recommended and proven to improve bone mineral density, and several promising new therapies on the horizon. In a 2021 review of the literature, all bisphosphonates appeared to be effective in reducing the incidence of vertebral fractures compared with placebo.[199] Both zolendronate and denosumab are more powerful agents and have been proven to be more effective than bisphosphonates for fracture risk reduction. Similarly, anabolic agents such as romosozumab, abaloparatide, and teriparatide are more effective than bisphosphonates for fracture risk reduction. As such one recommendation reported in *Bone Reports* in 2021 recommended either zolendronate, denosumab, or an anabolic agent for patient at "high or imminent risk" for fracture.[43]

10 Osteoporotic Compression Fractures

Spinal compression fractures are fractures of the vertebral body, which is the major load-bearing component of the spine. It is important to specify that these are spinal osteoporotic compression fractures, and not just spinal compression fractures, because there are many other causes of compression fractures, and their underlying causes are much different. The discussion of all compression fractures in general would include at a minimum, the topics of metastatic cancer and trauma, which requires an entirely different approach. Books about urgent and emergent issues would not seem practical, and needless to say, there is no time to consult a medical reference in an emergency.

And for the avid reader with a love for reading and an encyclopedic memory, many of the same multivolume references used by physicians and surgeons can be purchased online in the present day, should they have no problem with the cost, which is prohibitively expensive for many. One challenge to patients today is the vast amount of material made available but lacking any frame of reference. Eliminating the many causes of compression fractures will serve the interest of the majority of the audiences seeking this book.

There is not enough time in the day to inform oneself of all of the many causes of compression fractures. The treatments differ greatly or are oversimplified, and will give the reader an incorrect picture of treatment options for them. For example, someone with a compression fracture due to a metastatic lesion may or may not be a candidate for radiation treatment. There is no discussion of the management of cancer in the present book. Additionally, in reference to causes of compression fractures that are due to other underlying processes, chronic loss of BMD makes the treatment of that problem so much more complex and increased the chances of a worse outcome.

There are numerous causes of compression fractures and their treatments, and should not be worked up without the aid of a physician. These compression fracture become increasingly more common, later in life. Why are they more common later in life? That is because our bone quality deteriorates as we get older. In some patients, this can reach a critical level. This most often is due to osteoporosis, which is a state of low bone density meeting a defined measurement threshold. If the underlying cause of compression fractures are not addressed, just treating them as they occur will result in more fractures, chronic pain, disability due to spinal deformity, and ineffective treatments (see figure below).

Multiple Osteoporotic Compression Fractures with a Resulting Spinal Deformity

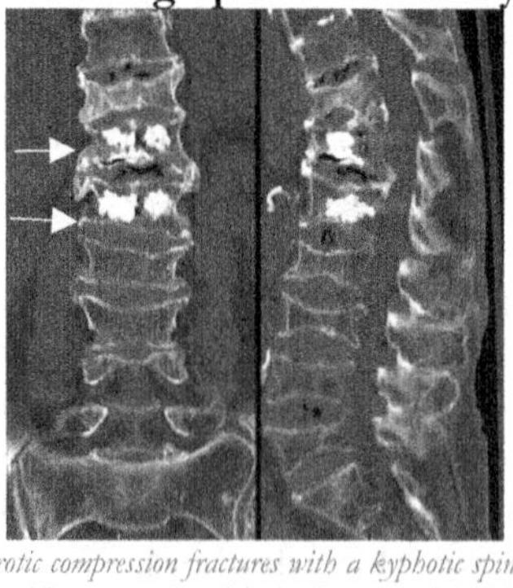

Figure 21. Osteoporotic compression fractures with a kyphotic spinal deformity in an 80 year-old woman, CT scan. Coronal Reconstruction of the lumbar spine (left), Note at T12 and L1 (arrows) the presence of prior cement treatment. Due to the worsening and untreated osteoporosis, subsequent fractures have occurred at every level, resulting in thoracolumbar kyphosis (image, right).

Acute Osteoporotic Compression Fracture of the Second Lumbar Vertebra

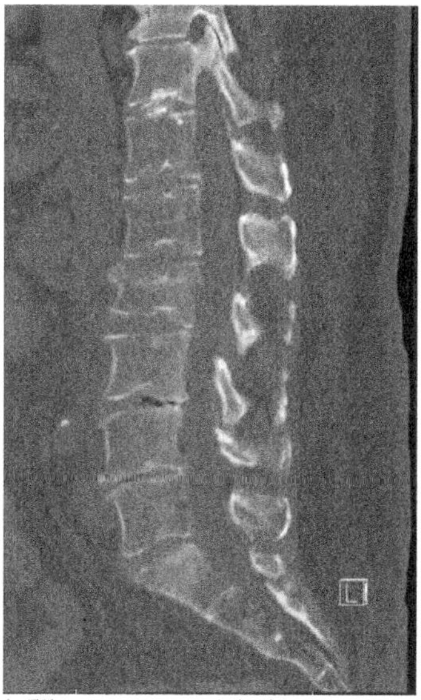

Figure 22. Sagittal CT reconstruction of the lumbar spine, showing an acute L2 compression fracture. There is a significant loss of bone density evident. This patient has a previous diagnosis of osteoporosis.

It is estimated that the cost of treatment for compression fractures amount to roughly $1 billion a year in the United States. The vast majority of compression fractures do not require any surgical intervention, or invasive treatment for the patient to achieve adequate pain relief. They are most commonly located in the 'thoracolumbar' spine (often referred to as thoracolumbar, especially when referring to the segments T10, T11, T12, L1, or L2, or T10-L2 in short). Often, patients obtain significant pain relief, with over the counter analgesic medication such as anti-inflammatories, avoiding strenuous labor, bracing, and obtaining a workup to evaluate for osteoporosis and other potential underlying conditions.

One's peak bone mass occurs at the age of 20-30. As with many lifetime processes, it is thought that there is a genetic influence which can impact the rate of this bone mass change.

Certain variables are thought to influence peak bone mass, including but not limited to nutrition, repetitive and chronic weightbearing, hormone influence and drug exposures such as glucocorticoids as mentioned above. Glucocorticoid/steroid use is particularly worrisome because it results in early-onset osteoporosis, and any chronic use needs observation at the discretion of a healthcare expert.

After the peak bone massed is reached at approximately age 30, it begins to slowly decline. Estrogen deficiency can result in rapid bone loss. Other exposures as well. While women can experience osteoporotic fractures in their 60s, this does typically does not occur in men until their 70s. However, some evidence points to men having a slightly higher likelihood of spinal osteoporotic fractures then women beginning in the 40s.

11 Bracing

The use of a spinal brace, in this book, is occasionally defined as an orthosis, or an external orthosis. For the spine, a thoracolumbar and cervicothoracic brace limits but does not completely restrict motion principally in 4 directions at the junction between the regions of the cervical, thoracic, and lumbar spine. These four directions are forward, backward, and side-bending (flexion, extension, and lateral bending). The goal of this type of bracing is generally to aid with pain and not to stabilize. This assistive device appears to help some patients with reducing acute back pain after a compression fracture. It does not appear to aid with radicular pain, a lancinating electric-shock feeling, often with associated tingling, that radiates from the back outward. Radicular pain is worrisome for nerve root compression.

A back brace, or neck brace, is an externally applied device to "strengthen or support" a body part. The function of these braces is theoretically to restrict motion, limit pain, prevent worsening spinal deformity, and to facilitate healing. Opponents of bracing argue that the quality of the medical evidence used to justify bracing for compression fractures is substandard.

Often, a patient may ask if bracing is absolutely necessary. This is not an unusual question. However, to answer this question, one must define the goal of bracing and answer the question in the context. A more rigid brace is often prescribed to a patient with the hopes that it will increase the likelihood that a compression fracture will heal, limit pain, and perhaps increase the chances of bone healing overall, as well as encourage the rapid healing of bone, and even prevent a postural deformity (kyphosis), which is a common cause of a major debilitating spinal imbalance.

And so, for those arguing that the evidence for the use of a brace is not strong, the risks are very low. When recommended for acute pain, thoracolumbar bracing has no match when patients ask what options they have, so as to avoid pain medication, some of which can lead to potential addiction.

Indeed, many of the challenges of medicine arise from demonstrating that an intervention may cause a benefit. It has been discussed the challenges in osteoporosis, in how to demonstrate a small improvement while isolating the numerous causes of osteoporosis. When evaluating the effectiveness of bracing on fracture healing, would one expect bracing to cause the fracture to heal faster? If so, how much faster? There is no evidence that bracing accelerates fracture healing, but if it did, this effect might be very small and difficult to detect without a very large study. Patients with compression fractures often do not begin treatment of the underlying cause of underlying osteoporosis within the first few months that bracing is recommended. And in others, they begin during the observation period. This variation further clouds the ability to detect a small difference between the treatments.

Another fundamental issue is present. To demonstrate a small change, two groups of patients at a minimum should be studied- those with and those without the intervention being studied. The patients without an intervention are known as the control population. There are very few effective pain reduction options, many patients will not want to participate in a study such as this. Designing a study that limits observational errors and bias is very difficult, and most often, a study cannot be free of design flaws. So these represent barriers to researching spinal bracing for compression fractures— limiting the number of studies that show effectiveness at accelerating fracture healing, as well as limiting pain.

Proposed Rationale For The Use of Spinal Bracing For Osteoporotic Compression Fractures

Promote Spinal Healing
Prevent Spinal Deformity
Decrease Deformity Growth
Limit Pain
Limit Range of Motion- Prevent Exacerbation of Injury

*Table 5 Rationale For The Use of Spinal Bracing for Osteoporotic Compression Fractures. *While the mechanism of a spinal brace is to limit range of motion, this limitation is often helpful for younger patients who need a reminder to limit potentially injurious activity shortly after a recent compression fracture.*

Variations in Bracing Protocols

Limited research leads to informal bracing protocols and institutional variation. The effectiveness of bracing in preventing worsening compression fractures, ie. deformity, or to prevent new compression fractures (which also cause deformity), has not been well demonstrated. In the US, bracing is a very common practice, as potential risks of treatment are limited. Chronic use of bracing can cause muscle atrophy and pressure ulcers, a risk that would be expected to increase with time. Again, as compared with the overall number of treatments available to patients with compression fractures, the profile is favorable. Essentially, there are not too many non-invasive treatments for acute compression fracture pain.

When a compression fracture is very severe, defined as debilitating and unrelenting pain, postural deformity, and even resulting in neurological deficits such as weakness— the treatment is often some variation of a surgical or interventional procedure.[14] First, not all patients are the same, and not all fractures are the same and these treatments are all administered on an individual basis.

Bracing Limits Motion of The Spine

Bracing is thought to limit pain by limiting flexion of the trunk. Flexion is a forward bending motion, which naturally places increased mechanical stress on the vertebral body. In the case of a recent compression fracture, this increased mechanical stress would be expected to increase pain, and potentially cause further worsening of the vertebral compression fracture.[200]

Medical Evidence – Bracing of Osteoporotic Compression Fractures

Reviews of medical studies for osteoporotic compression fractures finds contradictory conclusions ranging from a significant benefit to none at all. Again, that all depends on the outcome studied. Most recently, in *Global Spine Journal*, a systematic review of 4 randomized clinical trials and 3 prospective cohort studies found generally helpful evidence:

> "The use of spinal orthoses in neurologically intact elderly patients aged 60 years and older with osteoporotic compression vertebral fractures **results in improved biomechanical vertebral stability, reduced kyphotic deformity, enhanced postural stability, greater muscular strength and superior functional outcomes."[200] (emphasis added)**

[14] See surgical procedures Chapter for more details.

Potential Adverse Effects of Bracing

It is not commonly known that wearing a spinal brace may be associated with possible adverse effects.[201] However, increased discomfort may not be thought of as an adverse effect, but technically, if a patient experiences increased pain due to the brace, or develops breakdown of the skin due to constant daily pressure (pressure ulcer) then these are technically an adverse event of spinal bracing. One can infer that the overall risks of bracing is very low, as they can all be obtained over-the-counter— that is, without a prescription. Note that neck bracing carries the added risk of potentially increasing difficulty with swallowing food or liquids (see table below).

Abbreviated List of Known Adverse Effects of Spinal Bracing for Osteoporotic Compression Fractures

Pressure ulcers
Increased pain
Trouble Swallowing
Nerve Palsies
Skin Rashes

Types of Spinal Braces

There are many types of braces, for a variety of indications, and only those that are pertinent to fractures will be discussed. Many of the variations in bracing are designed for scoliosis, which is beyond the scope of this discussion. Many patients with compression fractures have longstanding scoliosis, which may prevent comfortable bracing to be applied. Custom bracing for this should be measured and applied by an expert with experience with scoliosis due to the potential risk to make scoliosis worse, or cause increased pain due to an improperly fitting brace. Further confusing the picture are the number of names referring to the same types of braces.

Ultimately the decision-making process for the brace that is recommended to treat a compression fracture is dependent upon the location of the fracture and the familiarity that the prescriber has with them, and what is available, which in many hospitals is limited.

12 Bone Stimulators

Since 1841, physicians and scientists have been experimenting with ways to accelerate fracture healing with reports on success with treatment of a tibial fracture.[202] Bone growth stimulators, are devices worn around the region of a fracture, in a similar manner to a brace whereby the electric circuit within the device induces an electromagnetic field that is believed to stimulate bone growth. This is also known as electronic bone growth stimulation (EBGS). There are generally several categories of electromagnetic fields generated: direct current stimulation (DCS), capacitive coupling electric fields (CCEF), and pulsed electromagnetic fields (PEMF).[15] Overall, these all refer to types of EBGS. As the name implies, direct current stimulation provides direct current to the operative site by implantable positive and negative leads, attached to the implantable battery. This may be kept permanently to avoid a second surgery just for retrieval of the battery and leads. Overall, due to major improvements in implants, and other technologies that encourage fusion, the DCS battery and leads are not commonly utilized, and only under certain circumstances, such as a failure of fusion. In CCEF, the leads are placed across the fusion site, above the skin and patients are encouraged to wear these for as much as possible, even 24 hours. PEMF is also known as therapeutic magnetic resonance and requires less use, typically between 3-8 hours per day. However, this therapy is considered experimental and investigational for most

---

[15] There are many more types of electromagnetic fields. As experimental evidence is identified in the laboratory setting, other avenues of potential benefit under this category of treatment. However, nearly all categories are considered experimental and investigational in the area of spinal fractures. Understanding the evidence for EBGS as a nascent group of treatments for spinal fractures is important as these are nonetheless marketed towards patients.

indications by many insurance carriers (eg., Aetna[203]) including the prevention and management of osteoporosis. Similarly, Medicare has set strict criteria for coverage of EBGS, particularly limited to certain spinal fusions. EBGS are not covered by Medicare for the healing of spinal fractures.[204]

DCS is unique in that it is an implanted battery system. In any case, someone with a lumbar spine fracture they must be treated surgically for a fracture to be a candidate for DCS. The bone growth stimulator does not cause pain or any symptoms, keeping in mind that if it is used after a spine fracture, or even after a surgery to stabilize the spine after a fracture, a spinal surgery requiring screws, rods, and other stabilizing implants, symptoms from DCS would often not be detectable due to masking of the pain from normal postoperative pain and discomfort. DCS is most often reserved for patients with pseudoarthrosis requiring reoperation to correct a failed fusion.

What does the bone growth stimulator do anyway? A number of laboratory findings (in vitro) suggest that intracellular calcium and a whole host of other factors (eg. fibroblast growth factors, osteocalcin, and alkaline phosphatase) are thought to be increased during the process of bone healing.[205]

Overall, there are a number of different systems, and a growing body of evidence exists supporting the idea that improved fusion rates can occur with the use of these bone growth stimulators. Also, growing evidence suggests that EBGS are helpful after spinal compression fractures, albeit there is much less evidence to justify the expense. Lastly, these tools will be reviewed below in terms of their utility after spinal fusion surgery.

Does Electronic Bone Growth Stimulation Lead to Spinal Healing after a Compression Fracture?

There are certain instances where EBGS may potentially aid with fracture healing. However, EBGS is not a standard treatment for compression fractures due to the lack of evidence.

Fundamentally, bone growth stimulation is less likely to be of benefit when there is a substantial gap between the two fracture surfaces. Therefore, when discussed in the following section in the scope of fusion surgery, one of the principles of fusion surgery is just that, to avoid gaps where growing bone cannot span— That is one purpose of bone grafting.

So far, there is not any evidence that suggests that EBGS makes compression fracture healing worse. However, without any satisfactory evidence of benefit, this is a very expensive out of pocket treatment. For these reasons, physicians are not routinely providing EBGS for spine fractures.

The bulk of medical evidence for the clinical use of EBGS pertains to long bone fractures. Long bone fractures also benefit from a greater variety of options including ultrasonic osteogenesis stimulators— devices that stimulate healing with ultrasound, which is covered by many insurance carriers for a variety of fracture types. The spine is biomechanically much different and it will be a matter of time before this technology is perfected to the point that a benefit is demonstrated and they are recommended.

Does Electronic Bone Growth Stimulation Help for Healing After a Spinal Surgery?

Unlike compression fractures, evidence suggests that EGBS may help with fusion surgery, particularly in osteoporotic patients, which has led to the routine recommendation of EGBS for higher risk fusion surgeries. Fundamentally, there are major challenge to fusion surgery in the setting of osteoporosis. For one, spinal hardware such as pedicle screws require solid bone to maintain bone purchase, maintain spinal alignment, prevent loosening, and to keep the spine immobilized— a requirement for bone to grow across the fused segment. The hardware, for example, a titanium alloy, is able to handle the stress and fatigue of the body, for approximately a year, potentially longer. If the body does not fuse before then, reliance on this titanium implant as an internal brace for distribution of the load of the body weight, through repetitive cycles of flexion and extension can lead to fractured titanium rods, screws, or in the case of osteoporotic bone, the hardware may loosen, causing debilitating pain— requiring reoperation.

Spinal hardware does not work so well in the setting of osteoporosis. Similarly, when a bone graft or cage made of plastic polymer or metal is placed in a disc space, to restore alignment and decompress nerves, if the adjacent bone in contact is soft, the implant will not do its job properly. What happens is that the implant will settle into the endplates, losing that restoration of alignment, and losing the indirect decompression of the nerve roots.

One analogy for osteoporosis and implants is that of placing a screw in sheetrock versus the wooden stud. Very osteoporotic bone is often described as an egg shell. In osteoporosis, the cortical bone on the surface of the spine is thins like the calcium in an eggshell— apart from the shell, there is no other substrate for the screw to obtain fixation. There is even a great chance that this cortical surface can break, providing no surface for fixation. In extreme instances, technologies such as acrylic cements have to be injected through screws to maintain a modicum of fixation strength, which greatly increases surgical complexity. And without bone, even cement can become loose. Most of the fixation strength of a screw comes from a long course through the spinal segment, with well-mineralized trabecular bone of adequate density.

Regarding the EBGS literature pertaining to healing after spinal surgery, it is again important to understand that that the research is very limited. One recommendation published in 2014 by Kaiser et al. was only for direct current stimulation (DCS) to be used, which is an intraoperative implant placement and not to be worn on a brace.[206] These leads would then be attached to an internal battery source in a separate incision and the lead is tunneled from the operative site to the internal battery, similar to a pacemaker or spinal cord stimulator. The use of EBGS has been demonstrated narrowly following spinal lumbar fusion surgery in patients under the age of 60, whereas over the age 60, no benefit was observed. One can also infer from those osteoporotic patients, being predominantly over 60, would be unlikely to derive a benefit for EBGS after spinal fusion surgery.

In another small study, pulsed electromagnetic field stimulation appeared to provide a benefit, but the authors in the aforementioned guidelines paper could not recommend for or against PEF due to the limitations of the study design. However, for the interested reader, in 1990, 195 patients were randomized to PEMF stimulation, or to bracing along, where 92% of PEMF stimulation achieved fusion success versus 65% with bracing alone, which on the surface appeared to be major difference.[207] In another study, PEMF was reserved for 100 patients who had failed fusion and became symptomatic with pain at an average of 9 months after fusion surgery. After PEMF application for 2 hours a day for the following 3 months, two-thirds of patients achieved fusion with a pain reduction.[208] These results are promising, especially for these adjuncts that have a very low risk profile. Perhaps, after high-quality studies are conducted, additional EBGS technologies can be applied to fracture healing.

13 Vertebroplasty

Often, compression fractures can cause pain that does not improve with time, or with most noninvasive treatments. Or, the pain is too severe from the point of onset, that debilitating back pain prevents one from performing their daily routine. In other words, their activities of daily living. In some instances, acute pain may become so severe, leading to insomnia. For many others, the concern is that prolonged narcotic requirements will result in addiction.

The severe pain of a compression fracture may take weeks, or even months to subside, in those where they occur. According to some estimates, up to 40% of patients with compression fractures may require additional care for persistent pain attributed to compression fractures.[209]

The Natural History of Painful Compression Fracture in A Selection of Recent Clinical Studies

Author	Study (Year)	Natural History
Voormolen[210]	VERTOS I (2007)	Approximately 20% of patients developed chronic low back pain.
Ploeg[211]	Review of Clinical Studies (2006)	Approximately 20% with persistent pain.
Klazen[212]	Prospective Study (2010)	33% with pain treated at 2 years with prescription analgesics and physical therapy.
Venmans[213]	VERTOS II (2012)	40% requiring prescription analgesics at 1 year.

Table 6. Selection of Studies. Long term outcomes after osteoporotic compression fracture in patients who were not treated with vertebroplasty.

Looking at the brief list of studies above, the natural history of compression fractures is one of chronic pain. There are numerous identified causes of chronic pain after a compression fracture. The key time point at which the acute pain of a compression fracture may transition to long term, chronic pain is unknown, but has been highlighted in some studies, such as at 3 months in the VERTOS II study by Venmans et al.[214]

Common Identified Causes of persistent pain after a compression fracture

Incomplete healing/ nonunion (fracture does not heal)
Spinal deformity / Imbalance
Pseudoarthrosis (fracture not healing after a surgery)
Nerve Root Injury
Opiate-induced hyperalgesia

While some of the above causes of chronic pain will be discussed in their appropriate sections of this book, a detailed review of some of these causes are out of the scope of this discussion. Briefly, when a compression fracture occurs, inflammation within the bone triggers a release of inflammatory markers which is accompanied by pain. Pain fibers within the bone are thought to be stimulated by local injury and also by any movement. Shortening of the vertebral body can cause painful nerve compression directly or indirectly, spinal deformity which causes a painful shift forward of the center of gravity, which causes muscle and joint pain from overuse of spinal muscles and other joints to realign the body over the favored center of gravity. Chronic narcotic use can exacerbate the pain, a condition referred to as opiate-induced hyperalgesia (OIH).[215] This condition has been more clearly observed in abdominal surgery patients in a study drawing a correlation between remifentanil (a potent intravenous opiate) and both increased postoperative pain and postoperative pain medication needs.[215] One of the difficulties with understanding how common OIH may be is the lack of a well-defined diagnostic criteria and lack of any objective confirmatory testing methods. Basically, this can be described as pain that generalizes to a broader area of the body and worsens substantially with rising opiate tolerance.

The Vertebroplasty Technique

In a vertebroplasty procedure, the technique is performed under sterile conditions. After conscious sedation or general anesthesia, the patient is placed prone on an operating table and his or her skin prepared and then draped in a sterile manner to limit the risk of infection. Infection is rare, but infection of PMMA cement is a devastating and challenging complication to manage due to the major difficulties with removal of infected cement. Following this, using fluoroscopic guidance (a type of portable x-ray machine), the spinal level of interest is located (see figure).

Vertebroplasty and Kyphoplasty: Transpedicular Approach

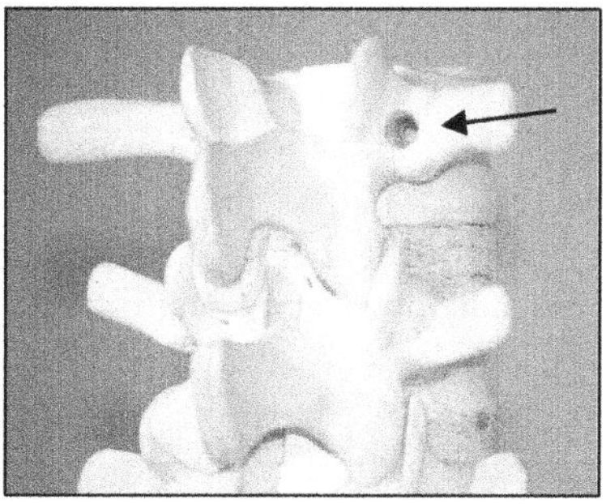

Figure 23. An illustration of the transpedicular approach, the anatomical corridor to the anterior vertebral body. The patient is lying face down on an operating table, and the initial entry is via a large bore needle overlying the spinal level of interest.

A metal cannula is guided through the pedicle, and into the vertebral bodies (See Figure below). The figure shown below utilizes a right and left pedicle entry, which is most often the case with kyphoplasty or other advanced techniques that attempt to restore the height of a vertebral body. Restoring only one side would place the patient at risk for scoliosis. However, occasionally, patients have compression fractures only on one side, which can cause scoliosis (also referred to as a coronal plane deformity). Scoliosis is not only a deformity involving abnormal kyphosis (bending or forward flexion), but a deformity in an imaginary plane intersecting at a right angle.

Vertebroplasty and Kyphoplasty Technique: Bilateral Transpedicular Cannulation of The Vertebral Bodies

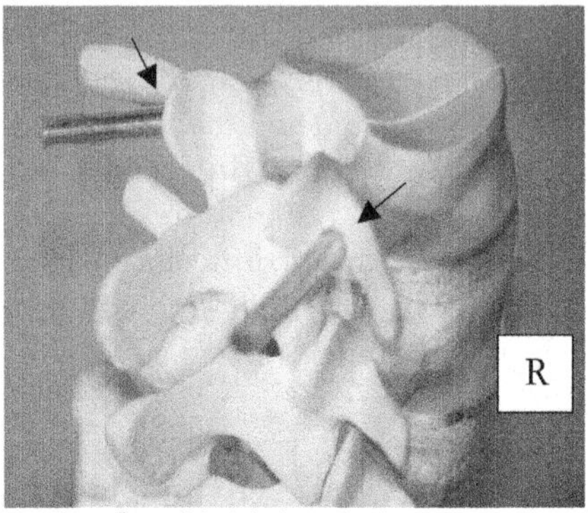

Figure 24. A Sawbones® model of the lower lumbar spine is shown (sawbones.com), posterolateral/oblique view showing brass pin placement in the right (R) and left pedicles of the third lumbar level (L3, arrows illustrating entry points of the L3 pedicles).

Centering the approach through the pedicles is performed in a variety of freehand or image-guided methods which is beyond the scope of this book.[16] Such as freehand a physician first guides a needle by x-ray through the posterior musculature and most commonly, through the pedicle, a bony bridge that leads to the vertebral body. Following confirmation that the syringes are in the appropriate anterior position of the vertebral body, a rapidly-setting plastic polymer is mixed, and after appropriate viscosity is obtained, it is injected through the cannula (shown in the figures as brass pins). The plastic polymer used is polymethylmethacrylate (PMMA), often referred to as cement, and is the same chemical compound in plexiglass.

---

[16] Several operative spinal surgery and neurosurgery manuals provide detailed descriptions of these techniques, available online for free or in print.

Potential Risks of Vertebroplasty

The use of fluoroscopy is critical during the injection of cement to ensure that the surgeon or interventionalist can ensure that the location of cement is known at all times, as it can happen that PMMA could begin to leave the vertebral body and enter veins, which is a risk for causing a pulmonary embolus, but also exiting the vertebral body in the direction of the spinal canal and vertebral foramen. A pulmonary embolus could occur when cement enters the veins and travels towards the lungs, blocking blood flow in a part of the lungs, preventing oxygen exchange, or worse.

Thankfully, a pulmonary embolus is relatively less common and the risk is further lowered by ensuring that the cement has hardened sufficiently before injecting into the vertebral body. Using more viscous PMMA is thought to similarly lower the likelihood of PMMA entering the veins and travelling towards the epidural veins which can fill the spinal canal and compress the spinal cord and nerves— this is a risk for paralysis both by the action of heat released by hardening cement, or by direct compression. Patients that have osteoporosis, and particularly severely decreased BMD may often have fractures of the posterior wall of the vertebral body that are poorly visualized and even the pedicle, which may not appear on imaging and constitutes a high risk. The PMMA could potentially extrude through these fractures (see figure).

Proximity of Pedicle Wall and Nerve Roots – A Risk for Extrusion of PMMA

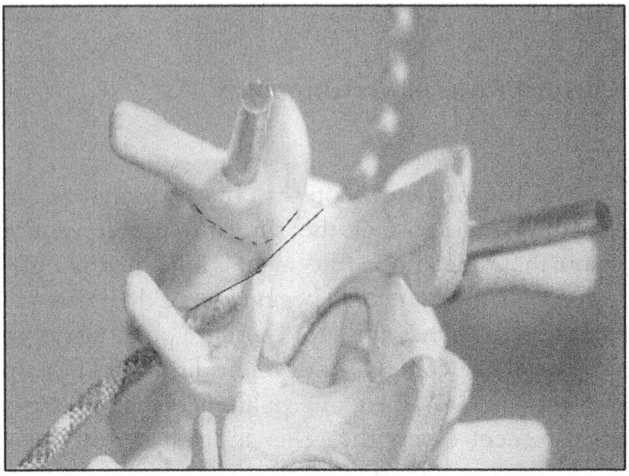

Figure 25. Spine model, posteroinferior view, illustrating a close relationship between pedicle cannulation tools for placing cement (brass pins), and the exiting nerve root (braided cable). The course of the nerve root (solid line) is close in proximity to the medial and inferior edge of the pedicle (dotted line).

As with every single step in any surgery or procedure, precision placement of the pedicle cannulation tool is essential. Often, very small pedicles can be a challenge to safe placement, and other approaches have been described to lower the chance that cement can extrude a pedicle and damage a nerve root. Also placement of the vertebroplasty further anterior from the posterior spinal canal may be an option. This is routinely performed in the case of a kyphoplasty, where elevating the anterior aspect (front) of the vertebral body will also maximize the improvement of the natural alignment.

Spinal Model after PMMA Vertebroplasty

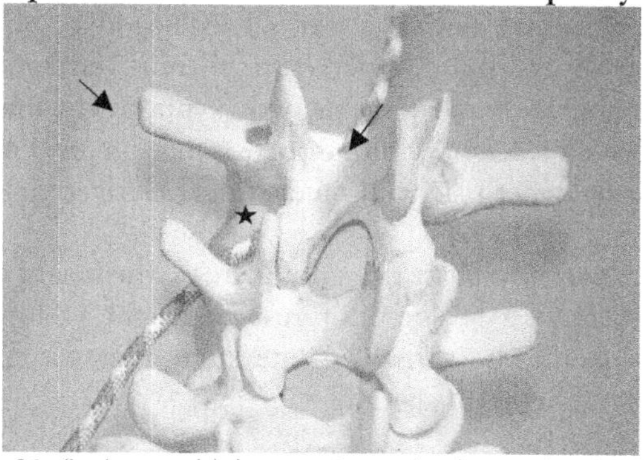

Figure 26. Sawbones model, demonstrating vertebroplasty, and residual PMMA can be seen, as illustrated by black arrows indicating gray cement at the site of pedicle entry. The L3 nerve roots exit just beneath the L3 pedicles (left L3 nerve root labelled by a star).

In some instances of severe pain without significant shortening of the vertebral body, a vertebroplasty results in immediate relief. The reason for this is that PMMA, during the course of hardening, will release heat and through direct toxicity, will damage small pain fibers within the vertebral body resulting in pain improvement. This may be reported as early as two hours after the procedure, usually after allowing for anesthesia to wear off.[216] Another mechanism where this occurs is thought to be through the limitation of motion of the compression fracture site, which most certainly would be expected to cause low back pain (referred to as mechanical pain— pain with body movement).

Kyphoplasty

The kyphoplasty utilizes the same approach as the vertebroplasty, and is a natural extension of the procedure. Often, in a compression fracture, there is vertebral body height loss, and in some patients, the kyphoplasty may potentially restore that height without open spinal surgery. Open surgery is vastly higher risk, with much longer recovery.

A vertebroplasty does not increase the height of a vertebral body, and so it does not restore height. However, it will subsequently be shown in one study that vertebroplasty can potentially correct alignment.

Kyphoplasty restores the height of the vertebral body, and hence, can decrease kyphosis and potential restore sagittal alignment. Sagittal malalignment most often causes a typing forward, and in the cause of compression fractures, is usually due to the combined effects of multiple compression fractures that each causes a cumulative effect on a hunched over posture. Kyphoplasty is limited in its deformity correction, and that is where one might have to consider major corrective spinal surgeries— this is especially in matters of spinal deformity surgery and nerve root compression. Due to the complicated decision-making process of open surgery with osteoporotic compression fractures, this discussion will be very limited—thankfully, relatively few patients will have to undergo open surgery.

In brief, in spinal surgery, when the term "surgical treatment" is used, it refers to spinal surgery, and not kyphoplasty or vertebroplasty. It is referred to as an intervention, or percutaneous intervention as the procedure is performed through a large bore needle, and not requiring an incision. The need for an incision is what defines "open" surgery generally, but there are exceptions to every rule.

Even this definition is changing, with the use of endoscopic spinal surgery of a spinal nerve root, followed by spinal stabilization with screws and rods (segmental fixation). Treatments that are performed through a large-bore needle (percutaneous) and are called interventional treatments. Two interventional treatments are vertebroplasty and kyphoplasty. The vertebroplasty procedure was first performed as early as 1984 for the treatment of a painful cervical vertebral hemangioma in a young woman.[217]

Indications

Referring to the table below of indications, these are reported for vertebroplasty, but generally include kyphoplasty as well. This is not a comprehensive list of indications as there are many pathologies not included in this book that are outside of the focus of this book. Kyphoplasty indications reflect an objective to restore vertebral body height. In review of the vertebroplasty indications, the reader will obtain a general sense of the clinical issues that may potentially improve from vertebroplasty. Regarding the first indication in the table, osteoporotic compression fractures comprise the vast majority of patients, although a formal diagnosis of osteoporosis is not necessary. Typically, some patients may have unrelenting back pain, and either x-ray or usually CT evidence of a compression fracture. However, in a small number of patients, there is persistent pain that prevents any ambulation or any relief at all. With the guidance of a physician or another healthcare provider, the patient may require further imaging with an MRI to evaluate for underlying disc herniations, stenosis, and evaluate for ligamentous injury which is not typically common. Fortunately, most patients do not have intractable back pain that does not respond to any medical treatment.

Indications and Contraindications for Vertebroplasty as Reported by Predley et al. in *American Family Physician*[218]

Potential Indications
Persistent Pain for Greater than 2 Weeks, Despite Nonsurgical Treatment for any Osteoporotic Cervical, Thoracic, or Lumbar Compression Fracture
Painful Vertebral Hemangiomas
Vertebral Osteonecrosis
Potential Contraindications
Osteoporotic compression fracture with improvement by less invasive means (eg. Bracing, medication, lifestyle modifications)
Untreated coagulopathy (eg. Continued use of anticoagulation such as warfarin)
Discitis/osteomyelitis (infection of the disc and vertebral body).
Nerve compression or canal compromise as a result of collapse of the vertebral body.
Chronic compression fractures.
Greater than 80-90% collapse of the vertebral body.

Table 7. Indications and Contraindications for Vertebroplasty. Summarized from American Family Physician in 2002. Note, indications for the treatment of malignancies are beyond the scope of this discussion and have been omitted.[219] Indications and contraindications are provided for general insight and are not meant as a rule to apply to all patient's, who are advised to seek and obtain individualized care from their physician or healthcare provider.

A Comment on The General Indications of Vertebroplasty and Kyphoplasty

Nonresponsive, osteoporotic vertebral compression fractures constitute the majority of instances for the use of vertebroplasty or kyphoplasty. However, the first use of vertebroplasty was for the treatment of a cervical vertebral hemangioma, as mentioned above. A hemangioma is most often a benign tangle of blood vessels, which in a study performed in Iran was incidentally diagnosed in 26.9% of 782 spinal MRI studies, of which there were multiple hemangiomas in 33%.[220] Indeed, this is an incredibly common problem. Most vertebral hemangiomas do not cause symptoms, ie., back pain. In a review of the literature of symptomatic hemangiomas requiring a surgical/interventional treatment, out of 47 articles only 197 cases were identified.[220] Symptomatic hemangiomas often show evidence on an MRI of inflammation around the margin of the hemangioma, and will demonstrate a tendency to grow, even causing erosion of the neighboring bone, or even nerve root compression. Open surgery is avoided as these neoplasms are made entirely of blood vessels, which can bleed uncontrollably. Instead, endovascular treatment has had success with injection of materials that clot off the hemangiomas, materials such as polyvinyl alcohol, embolic materials such as glue, microparticle beads, or even the use of vertebroplasty/kyphoplasty with PMMA cement injection. Of those treated in the abovementioned series, 84% of subjects had complete relief in their symptoms. In another series, hemangiomas treated with any of the above techniques, had clinical and neurological improvement at up to a five-year follow-up.[221]

The Vertebroplasty Experience At a Single Center, As Recounted Through One Thousand Consecutive Vertebroplasties

In a sample series by Layton et al., the results of 673 vertebroplasty sessions for 552 patients for a total of 1000 spinal compression fractures were reported. In this series, 84% were related to osteoporosis, whereas 11% were treated for cancer, and 5% were treated for hemangioma and trauma.[222] Only 12% required general anesthesia, whereas nearly everyone else had conscious sedation, which is anesthesia to varying degrees that maintains a fine balance between reduced awareness of the surgery and limited pain while maintaining the ability to protect the airway and avoid a breathing tube that is required in general anesthesia (ie. intubation). The frequency of patient's requiring general anesthesia has steadily dropped over time. **For the majority of patients, pain levels reported, as recorded on a visual analogue scale, as compared with before surgery,**

saw a dramatic decrease pain just 2 hours post-surgery (see Figure Below).

Vertebroplasty For Osteoporotic Compression Fractures that Fail Medical Management Provides Improvements In Pain At Up to 2 Years, in a Series of 1000 Consecutive Treatments[223]

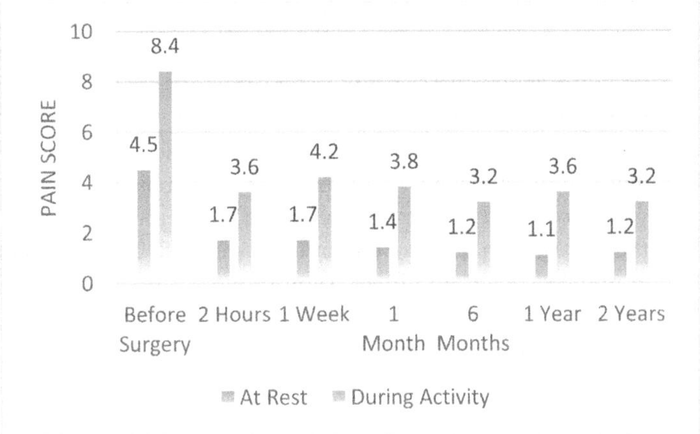

Figure 27. Vertebroplasty Improvement in a Series of 1000 Vertebroplasties. Pain Score is based on a numerical grading scale, called the visual analog scale (VAS).

It appears that in this series, most patients improved. How is it that summaries of the literature are less clear than this publication on demonstrating positive results? It is important to keep in mind that with single-center studies, the treatment outcomes tend to provide more optimistic outcomes. Anecdotally, Bafeta and co-investigators compared single-center to multi-center studies in 292 randomized clinical trials that compared treatment outcomes for total of 177 single center and 115 multi-center studies.[218] They found that on average, single-center trials showed a greater treatment effect than multi-center trials. In other words, a greater treatment effect may be expected from a single center, and one can surmise that a single center aggregating their data may be less apt to share their data in a study if their outcomes were below average. Bellomo opines in *Critical Care Medicine* that treatment guidelines should rarely be based on single-center outcomes, and his synopsis is rather decisive and worth sharing for the reader:

> "Many positive single-center trials have been contradicted when tested in other settings and, in one case, the subsequent definitive multicentered trial has found a previously recommended intervention associated with active harm. Problems inherent in the nature of single-center studies make recommendations based on their results ill advised. Single-center studies frequently either lack the scientific rigor or external validity required to support widespread changes in practice, and their premature incorporation into guidelines may make the conduct of definitive studies more difficult."[218]

Studies are More Than "Positive or Negative"

While Bellomo's aforementioned critique of single-center studies appears to settle the matter, others argue for a more nuanced approach to studies. Pocock and Stone argue to avoid the tendency to oversimplify a study into a "yea or nay" approval and to carefully examine study design.[224] When a study is said to support a treatment outcome, how much of a positive benefit does it provide to the patient? In other words, if an improvement is said to be significant, is it clinically significant? Most often, researchers use the term significant because they have determined that the results are statistically significant, and more likely a result of the intervention (eg. The Vertebroplasty) than a chance occurrence. To the dismay of many, a significant improvement does not guarantee that the magnitude of improvement is large enough to provide a noticeable difference for the patient. So, with regards to Pocock and Stone, details of a study matter, and not just the "positive or negative" finding of the effect of the treatment.

Understanding Clinically Important Differences

The "minimal clinically important difference" (MCID) is the term researchers use to describe the smallest improvement needed in a grading scale for a patient to achieve a noticeable difference. The MCID is specific to different grading scales. So, if five different grading scales were used in a study, and patients had "significant" improvements in these grading scales after a particular treatment, the reader would have to know if this was noticeable to the patient, viz. not just the statistician. In one study, the authors estimated the MCID for VAS to be three.[225] To complicate matters further, this MCID was in a study of acute pain which was not specific to any particular disease process, and in the emergency department.

The MCID will always differ, as there is no consensus as to how the MCID is calculated. There are two general methods of MCID calculation, relying on a prior reference range of values, or the MCID is a calculation derived from a specific study, which seems to be a prevailing method, and specific to each study.[226] To use an example for the cervical neck pain, in one specific study, the MCID (VAS-neck pain) ranged from 0.4 to 2.1, substantially less than in the general study.[227]

Returning to the figure describing the two-year outcomes of vertebroplasty interventions for 1000 consecutive vertebroplasties, VAS scores at rest and during activity were 4.5 and 8.4, respectively, immediately after surgery they were 1.7 and 3.6, and two-years following treatment they had improved further to 1.2 and 3.2, respectively. Therefore, with an immediate postoperative improvement of 2.8 at rest and 4.8 during activity, the immediate difference after surgery may not be noticeable, despite what it would seem in the figure above. However, by 2 years, this improvement after two years was 3.3 and 4.8 at rest and during activity respectively, which based on a single study where MCID was 3.0, the improvements would eventually be noticeable.

Proponents of this study may argue that while the immediate improvement was borderline at rest, the improvement with activity was substantial. Overall, after two years, the patient has improved to a VAS of 1.2 and 3.2 after two years, can it be assumed that this was the work of the vertebroplasty? That cannot be answered. The authors conclude their paper,

> "On the basis of our results, percutaneous PMMA vertebroplasty is a safe and effective method to treat vertebral compression fractures."[228]

"Safe and Effective" Studies Require a Control Population

However, there is one element lacking in this study that prevents the authors from making the popular statement above, ostensibly confirming that the study confirms that the treatment is safe and effective. However, to do so requires a population of patients that did not receive the vertebroplasty for comparison of effect (ie. the control group). There is no frame of reference otherwise. And while many studies that lack a control population may discuss how the results of the study compare to the natural history *reported in previously published studies*, the control population must be as similar to the study population in terms of characteristics (e.g. age, % female, etc.).

The American Psychological Association defines treatment efficacy in their "Criteria Evaluating Treatment Guidelines" as well as discussing some noteworthy pitfalls:

> "...How well does the intervention work?... The term *treatment efficacy* refers to a valid ascertainment of the effects of a given intervention as compared with an alternative intervention or with no treatment, in a controlled clinical context. The fundamental question in evaluating efficacy is whether a beneficial effect of treatment can be demonstrated scientifically...It is important to distinguish between the context of discovery of an intervention and the context of verification of its clinical efficacy. Historically, some interventions that were later proven by systematic evaluation to be very powerful have arisen from clinical innovations and case studies. The question of whether particular interventions have beneficial effects is best answered using research methodologies that have been refined over many years to reduce the uncertainties inherent in subjective judgment

> alone and to increase confidence in the strength of the intervention. The systematic application of these research strategies also promotes the welfare of patients.
>
> Without evidence of efficacy, health care professionals are forced to rely exclusively on their direct experience of the effects of different interventions — an approach that risks erroneous conclusions. **For example, in some cases, disorders resolve themselves without formal treatment; an intervention that had coincidentally been applied in such a case might erroneously be judged effective.** Some medical and psychological practices that initially appeared helpful and became widely accepted were subsequently found ineffective or even harmful."[229] (emphasis in bold)

Returning once again to the series of 1000 vertebroplasties— in the long run, the authors may be correct in their assertion that vertebroplasty is effective, the only issue is that their study lacks the required comparative population to demonstrate their claims. After all, the conclusions of a study should be derived from the collected evidence therein.

The Natural History of an Osteoporotic Compression Fracture

The natural history refers to the course of disease, progressing from onset to resolution, without treatment. And of course, upon deeper analysis, there is no absolute definition when one cannot agree when a disease actually began and what treatments just exactly may or may not impact the course of the disease. For the purpose of our discussion, the natural history of an osteoporotic compression fracture is observed only in a patient who has not received a vertebroplasty or other treatment physically altering the natural course. A review of the aforementioned table in this chapter shows that a substantial percentage of patients with osteoporotic compression fractures may experience chronic pain. However, how does the natural history fare when compared to vertebroplasty? The reader may be surprised to find that patients with a compression fracture undergo a dramatic improvement over 6 months without any treatment (See Figure Below).

Comparison of VAS Patient-reported Pain Scores in Three Clinical Trials Comparing Vertebroplasty to No Intervention Showing Early Improvement Regardless of Intervention

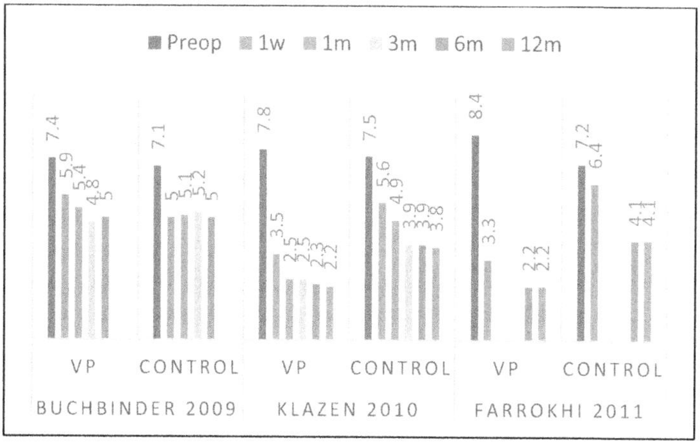

Figure 28 A Comparison of Vertebroplasty (VP) to Control Patients for the treatment of painful vertebral osteoporotic compression fractures in Three Clinical Trials: Buchbinder,[218] Klazen,[230] and Farrokhi[214]. Comparison is at set intervals: preoperatively (preop), 1 week (1w), 1, 3, 6, and at 12 months. Follow-up intervals differed between studies. Mean VAS scores are provided without standard deviation measurements.

In the aforementioned figure, it can be observed that both vertebroplasty (VP) and control patients alike experience substantial improvement. The study by Buchbinder in 2009 was significant in that both groups had similar improvements in pain at each interval and there was little if any difference to report whereas Klazen and Farrokhi found a substantial difference favoring vertebroplasty.

Kyphoplasty, Is it Superior to Vertebroplasty?

If the kyphoplasty is similar to a vertebroplasty, but involves a balloon to realign the height of the vertebral body, one would expect to find that the kyphoplasty is a superior procedure. However, the outcomes are very similar.

Potential Complications of Vertebroplasty or Kyphoplasty

For someone considering the vertebroplasty or kyphoplasty, this is an invasive procedure and the potential risks should be known. The risks between vertebroplasty and kyphoplasty are very similar, due to the similarities between approach, technique, and anatomy that the needle and cannula travel through on the route to the vertebral body. However, in one review of published studies, the authors found that the kyphoplasty was a safer procedure, with fewer reported adverse events.[214] This is not the same as stating that one procedure is safer than the other, as how a study defines a complication and the level of scrutiny and study design plays a major role in how many complications are reported or unreported, resulting in a number where there is no logical manner for which to draw comparisons to other studies with.

Even studies attempting to draw conclusions on the literature appear lack any degree of consistency. For example, in another review of the literature in 2015, Wang et al. found:

> "PKP[kyphoplasty] is superior to PVP[vertebroplasty] for the injected cement volume, the short-term pain relief, the improvement of short- and long-term kyphotic angle, and

lower cement leakage rate. However, PKP has a longer operation time and higher material cost than PVP."[231]

Overall, while there are benefits with both procedure, the kyphoplasty is designed to provide restore the height lost in from a compression fracture. This need may be addressed on an individual basis and should be a discussion between the patient and their spinal surgeon or treating interventionalist.

Abbreviated List of Reported Vertebroplasty Complications, As Compiled by the FDA

Infection	Neuropathy
Worsening of Fracture	Pedicle Fracture
Nerve Injury	Myocardial Infarction
Paralysis	Sciatica
Bleeding	Stroke
Allergy	Hypotension and Hypoxia
Pulmonary Embolus	Death

Table 8. Vertebroplasty Complications; a selection. A relatively more comprehensive list of potential complications may be found in medical device reports and other memoranda on the FDA website.[232]

Complications Pertaining to PMMA Cement

In terms of mechanical and chemical properties of materials used in spinal treatments, polymethylmethacrylate, or PMMA, also referred to as cement, is unique and warrants a more thorough review of its properties and its unique risk profile. Methylmethacrylate begins to rapidly link individual molecules after an accelerant is added, which is benzoyl peroxide. In this polymerization process, a significant amount of heat is released, which has been associated with a transient period of increased pain not lasting more than a few hours.[233] And so, PMMA has three mechanisms for nerve damage— heat damage, chemical damage, and physical compression.

As mentioned above, the placement of cement outside of the intended vertebral body, ie. extravasation of cement into the vicinity of a nerve, can causes irreversible nerve damage, chronic pain, and even paralysis. Fortunately, these events are rare, but are a devastating complication to be aware of.[234] These events seem to occur more frequently with malignancies and traumas with vertebral wall fractures, providing avenues of egress of the cement. These rare encounters are relevant to the focus of osteoporotic fractures, as the typical management of nerve compression is to surgically remove the cement mass through open surgery. Often, this requires a fusion with pedicle screw and rod placement, depending on if access to the cement requires the removal of enough stabilizing elements of the spine (such as the facet joints).

Moreover, procedural infections from vertebroplasty are rare, but are devastating. In one series, Park reported 3 cases out of 826(0.36%).[235] However, as "they" say, it is not rare if you are one of those (3 people), and in all 3 patients they underwent both open surgery and prolonged antibiotic treatment. However, 0.36% is not exactly a coin toss and some individuals are at higher risk for infection than others, usually from the same risk factors, such as poorly-controlled type II diabetes, and tobacco use.

Additional complications from PMMA use include temporary low blood pressure, due to chemical effects on the arteries,[236] as well as due to pulmonary embolism., which is the entry of fat from the vertebral marrow into the veins where it travels to the lungs. PMMA is very dense and will be easily distinguishable from fat when a CT scan is performed on the lungs,[237] whereas in fat embolism have been reported to result as a complication of vertebroplasty, diagnosed by MRI.[238] One other less discussed problem is local tenderness and pain, caused by cement exiting from the pedicle entry causing inflammation and tenderness due to irritation of the overlying muscles (see figure below).[239]

Backflow of Cement From Pedicle Entry Site

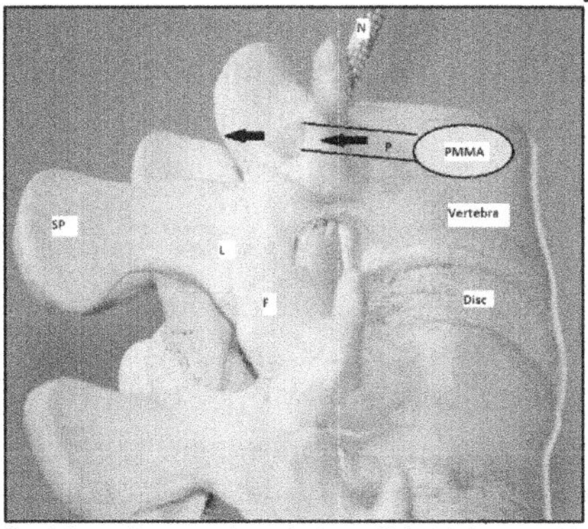

Figure 29. Backflow of cement through the pedicle (p) from a right-sided inferolateral view (from the right side). This backflow of cement (PMMA) from the vertebra can cause chronic muscle tenderness and back pain. Illustration Using Sawbones® Lumbar Spine Model. SP, spinous process; L: lamina; F: facet; Disc: intervertebral disc.

Kyphoplasty and Spinal Deformity Considerations

From the standpoint of spinal biomechanics, a compression fracture can initiate the vicious cycle of subsequent compression fractures caused by shortening of the anterior part of the spine. This initial shortening of the anterior vertebral body causes kyphosis, in other words, it is an exaggeration of the thoracic spine's normal curvature. This increased kyphosis makes matters worse by added stresses above normal, which can result in more shortening of the vertebral body. Indeed, it is a vicious cycle. While a vertebroplasty does not change spinal alignment, a kyphoplasty is a modified vertebroplasty whereby a balloon is inflated at the point where cement is normally injected in the vertebral body. The goal, would be to restore height to the vertebral body. Restoring height to the vertebral body can potentially help restore spinal alignment, or limit foraminal stenosis, which is the narrowing of the channel whereby paired nerve roots exit the spinal canal. Compression of these nerve roots eventually occurs with substantial collapse of a vertebral body, often greater than 50%. In other words, if the compression fracture has resulted in substantial shortening of the vertebral body, the inflated balloon can restore the height of the collapsing endplate. Then, a rapidly setting plastic polymer, polymethylmethacrylate, commonly referred to as cement, is injected into the spherical void created by the balloon.

Increasing thoracic kyphosis, usually at a point above 60 degrees as measured on a standing x-ray, will result in daily discomfort. The discomfort may be due to increased work of the spinal musculature (paraspinal muscles) as these muscles contract to offset the abnormal displacement of the upper body forward (see figure below).

Not everyone is a candidate for the kyphoplasty procedure. Often, the vertebral body cannot be restored in height with balloon inflation. This procedure can, and is frequently performed at different time intervals after a compression fracture. It is thought that partial healing of the fracture in the shortened position begins to occur after a week or two, and this can limit the extent that the vertebral body is restored to its original height.

How important is height restoration? That all depends on the patient. In one relatively larger study in 2019, 59 patients underwent one, two, or three level kyphoplasty between T5 and L5, whereby the authors sought to elucidate the relationship between height restoration and pain reduction. However, all patients improved in pain and none of the markers that were followed appeared to be significant factors in reducing pain.[240] In other words, it wasn't the anterior, middle, or posterior height improvements that were shown to lead to pain improvement. Most likely, it was the presence of the PMMA cement, which destroys nerve fibers carrying pain signals.

Spinal Compensation to Increased Kyphosis

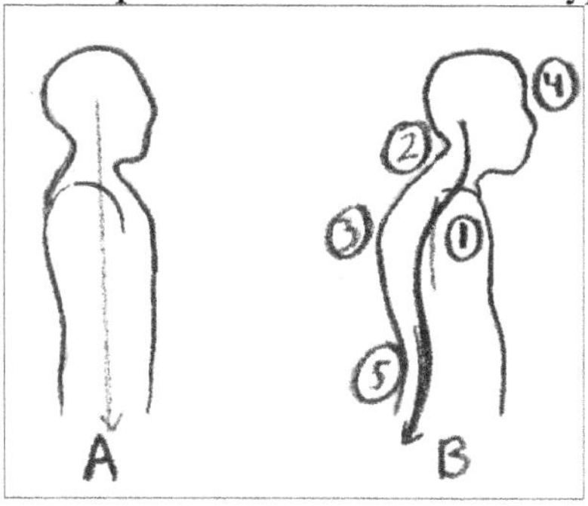

Figure 30 Kyphosis Development and Spinal Compensation. Ideal spinal alignment (A) is in a state of balance where the center of gravity (downward arrow) rests over the feet. Visible manifestations of increased kyphosis and a forward center of gravity include postural changes in the shoulders (1), neck extension (2), increased thoracic curvature (3) and increased extension of the low back (5). These maneuvers are aimed at maintaining horizontal gaze (4).

Joints throughout the body attempt to compensate for this increased thoracic kyphosis. Changes include extension of the cervical spine in the neck, extension of the low back (lumbar spine), and compensation via the pelvis, hip, knee, and ankles. Since the disk degenerates over time, it is normal for the balance of the spine to tip forward over time. By age 65, this balance can exceed parameters for an average person, without any back pain complaints, or known spinal problems.

If one's center of gravity is too far forward, then it becomes a laborious task to be balanced. That is where the term imbalance comes from. All of the joints in the body, along with supporting musculature are activated in an attempt to restore balance — ie., to prevent one from falling over. At this point, patients begin to struggle and a decrease in quality of life is observed. Nerve compression and back pain is

often relieved by leaning forward on a cane or walker, and that there is a relatively greater risk for the development of a compression fracture.[241] Most degenerative processes of the thoracic and lumbar spine result in an increase in kyphosis and pressure on osteoporotic bone.

Sagittal imbalance can be thought in other terms as a displaced center of gravity. This imbalance is almost always a forward displacement (termed, positive sagittal balance). Throughout life, the spinal discs degenerate, and one impact of this is a naturally increasing kyphosis throughout life, as observed in asymptomatic volunteer study participants.[242]

Studies Summarizing Vertebroplasty and Kyphoplasty

Cochrane is a UK-based research organization whose publications contain standardized reviews that summarize all relevant medical research in the pursuit of answering a research question. This organization has a reputation of high standards of conducting research. According to their review of vertebroplasties, their position on the use of vertebroplasty for the treatment of osteoporotic compression fractures is that their results of high-quality studies, most often consider a rigorous usually randomized clinical trials, vertebroplasty

The Benefits of Vertebroplasty and Kyphoplasty and Patient Satisfaction

In summary, if various medical review articles suggest that no obvious benefit in pain reduction can be demonstrated with vertebroplasty or kyphoplasty, why pursue a potentially life-threatening treatment? Unfortunately, this is an important question that there is no universal answer for. However, consider that out of a dozen patients considering this treatment, vertebroplasty or kyphoplasty, perhaps only two or three of them were satisfied with their improvement, and in another group of twelve patients, perhaps the majority were satisfied. Carefully consider the potential reasons that exist for variability in satisfaction, and the most important ones do not have to do with the surgical procedure itself.

In fact, the most important factor precedes the treatment itself, and it has to do with determining if your expectations align with that of your physician's. Setting expectations that are appropriate and understanding clearly what the physician considers a treatment success is also an important facet of informed consent. The word "successful" is often defined as meeting a "desired end".

Vertebral Body Stenting

Vertebral body stenting is a third generation procedure, separate from the vertebroplasty and kyphoplasty, and worthy of brief mention. A vertebral body stent works under the similar principle of an arterial stent. When people have narrowing of the arteries in their heart, the narrowing can be reopened by deploying a stent. A wire is navigated by x-ray to the location of the narrowing. When the stent is released from the wire, it is designed with sufficient force to open the artery to some degree. Sometimes, the vessels become calcified or are stiff from fibrous changes, or thickening of the vessel wall and a balloon can be expanded in the vessel first to open it up beforehand. After the balloon expands the vessel, the stent is deployed to hold the vessel open.

Now, with vertebral body stenting, balloon kyphoplasty occurs either before or after an expandable device is placed inside the vertebral body. With one system, a titanium stent is placed into the vertebral body, and then it is expanded with the force of a balloon in the manner that would be performed with a balloon kyphoplasty. As this stent is expanded open, it stays open and held in place by PMMA cement. In another iteration, the stented vertebral body is placed at the time of the kyphoplasty, the differences are minor.

Proponents of balloon kyphoplasty argue that the fracture fragments will realign when the vertebral body is restored to normal height. The process of restoration of the normal anatomical alignment, ie., away from the nerves and spinal cord, towards the normal alignment, is called ligamentotaxis.

Recollapse of the Vertebral Body After Kyphoplasty

This settling is problematic. Stenting of the vertebral body after kyphoplasty was designed to address this problem. The vertebral body can actually settle after the height is restored from a balloon kyphoplasty following a compression fracture. In a study of 203 patients who underwent kyphoplasty, 38.9% of patients suffered some measurable collapse of the vertebral body.[243] As with any study, it is important to consider the results of several studies as this figure of recollapse was reported by Heo and coinvestigators as only 3.21% (11 out of 343 patients).[244] Unfortunately, definitions and the timing vary between studies. There are several risk factors for recollapse of the vertebral body. In one review of the medical literature, five factors were identified as likely risk factors for recollapse. These risk factors included preoperative intravertebral cleft, presence of the compression fracture between T10 and L2, severe kyphosis, filling of cement in a "solid lump pattern", and patients with a higher than usual re-expansion of the vertebral body- which were all considered risk factors for some degree of recollapse.[245]

Risk Factors Associated with Recollapse After Vertebroplasty

Persistent Intravertebral Cleft[246]
Thoracolumbar Compression Fracture Level (T10-L2)[247]
Severe Kyphosis[245]
"Solid Lump" PMMA Filling Pattern[245]
Greater Vertebral Height Restoration[245]
Mid-Portion Type Fracture[248]
Involvement of Posterior Wall[248]

Intravertebral Cleft

There are numerous risk factors associated with recollapse. Perhaps the greatest risk is osteoporosis itself. The longer it goes untreated, the less likely anything will hold at the bone-cement interface at the microscopic level. In many instances, the PMMA injected can lose that interface that it develops and become a painful mass of what appears to be almost free-floating cement.

Often, with osteoporotic compression fractures, a gas-filled intravertebral cleft is identified, and it's presence on imaging is associated with pain, and also present in nearly half of patients.[249] The gas-filled cleft is thought to be the result of non-healing and some authors advocate for the filling of this cleft with PMMA cement during vertebroplasty, stating that there is a tendency for better outcomes when filled.[249]

Vertebral Stenting Does Not Provide Superior Results to Kyphoplasty

Now that the evidence is reviewed showing that the vertebral body often can recollapse after kyphoplasty, the argument has been made that a "structural support" could be deployed in the cavity formed after kyphoplasty in addition to cement placement. Again, vertebral stenting is a relatively newer technology and referred to as third generational vertebral augmentation, following cement delivery (1st gen), and then following balloon kyphoplasty (2nd gen.).[250] These devices invariably consist of a titanium expandable device and go by the proprietary names of Spine Jack® (Stryker Corp), OsseoFix® (Alphatec Spine, Inc.), and the Vertebral Body Stenting System® (Depuy Synthes Inc.). In all cases, they are inserted on both the right and the left side, as the concern is that, an expandable support on one side only could potentially cause scoliosis by uneven expansion of the vertebral body.

So far, there are very few clinical studies, and the majority of them find no additional benefit of vertebral body stenting over kyphoplasty. In a randomized clinical trial of 100 patients by Werner and co-investigators, the mean reduction of kyphosis was 4.5 and 4.7 degrees in kyphoplasty and vertebral body stenting, respectively.[251] Another trial, the SAKOS trial, compared Spine Jack ® vertebral body stenting to balloon kyphoplasty at 12 months, essentially finding no significant difference in the two.[252] The study was designed to study improvement in pain at up to 1 year after treatment, and there was no significant clinical difference reported, in other words, there was no difference in pain. Let's further examine the findings. Said the authors in their study:

> "The analysis…demonstrated the superiority of TIVAD[stent] over BKP[balloon kyphoplasty] ($p<0.0001$) at 6 months (88.1% vs. 60.9%) and at 12 months (79.7% vs. 59.3%)."

The authors stated that there was no difference in clinical improvement, and yet additional analysis showed that stenting was superior both at 6 months and at 12 months. Examining these claims further we read that,

> "Midline VB height restoration was more improved for TIVAD than for BKP at 6 months (**1.14**±2.61 mm vs. **0.31**±2.22 mm); $p=0.0246$) and 12 months after surgery (**1.31**±2.58 mm vs. **0.10**±2.34 mm; $p=0.0035$)."

Is 1.14 mm versus 0.31 mm a very big difference? Often researchers emphasize statistical findings, borderline statistical findings in this instance. But what is the context of this improvement? Is it known how much of a collapse occurred to begin with? Is it known what the height of the vertebral body is to begin with? The three most common levels treated in this study in descending order was L1, T12, and L2. Using a study of 100 cadavers as reference, for T12, the mean vertebral body height was 22mm measured in the front (anterior) and 29 mm measured in the back.[253] If the % height loss were estimated and the % of the vertebral height gain reported as well, we could truly get a sense of just how significant these results really are.

Let's further complicate the matter, and discuss that several authors have reported a height restoration with vertebroplasty as well, with average improvement in vertebral body height of 49% reported by Dublin,[253] 27% by Tang,[254] as well as significant height improvements reported by Chin[255] and Hiwatashi.[256] Proponents of newer devices that provide marginal, but greater improvements in spinal realignment will argue that shorter follow-up studies underemphasize the vital importance in maintaining appropriate spinal alignment. Abnormal spinal alignment, which can result from shortening of the disc space through disc degeneration as well as from compression fractures, can contribute to worsening spinal alignment and a reduction in quality of life. But at the present time, we are discussing what the current evidence can prove, and these devices are limited in long term studies.

> No statistically significant differences were shown between procedures for improvement in functional capacity and quality of life. Pain relief was significantly more marked in the TIVAD group compared to the BKP group at 1 month (p=0.029) and at 6 months (p=0.021) after surgery. No patient required surgical reintervention or retreatment at the treated level. No symptomatic cement leakage was reported. Adverse events were similar for both groups (41.2% in the TIVAD group and 45.2% in the BKP group). The incidence of adjacent fractures was significantly lower after the TIVAD procedure than after BKP (12.9% vs. 27.3%; p=0.043)."[257]

In a series of 20 patients with vertebral body stents, Muto reported a reduction in pain and good clinical outcomes at 12 months.[258] Very interestingly, "The height in the fractured vertebral body was increased in 12 of the 20 vertebral compression fractures (VCFs) by an average of 1.5 mm", which means that the vertebral body stenting did very little to restore height, or was used in the fashion of a kyphoplasty. In 32 patients with 46 treated VCFs, which included cases where bone collapse was caused by erosive metastatic cancer, a mean reduction in pain for most patients available at follow-up.[253]

Noticeably, the improvement in kyphosis improved by a mean 2 degrees difference only, which is fairly underwhelming and also may just reflect the variability seen during repeated measurements by the same physician, or by different physicians taking repeated measurements— there are at least four studies that demonstrate the high variability and inaccuracy when using this measurement (called the Cobb Angle).[259-262] In one case, there was re-collapse of the vertebral body. In one recent clinical trial, 300 patients were randomized to kyphoplasty or vertebral body stenting using The Spine Jack® device, which is shaped like a tire jack. Unfortunately, there is very little data to serve as an appraisal for long-term performance of vertebral body stenting in terms of preventing collapse of the vertebral body.

14 Spinal Surgery

Osteoporosis is a major risk factor for having a complication with spinal fusion surgery. A spinal fusion surgery (arthrodesis) involves the use of spinal fixation, ie., screws and rods, to stabilize one or more motion segments[17] of the spine. This subject is discussed in great detail in the author's books, *The Low Back Pain Guide* (2019), and *The Neck Pain Guide* (2020), where further information may be found.

When spinal surgery is required that involves the use of spinal implants such as screws and rods that immobilizes a spinal level, this is referred to as fusion surgery. When someone is "having a fusion" procedure, the actual fusion process occurs slowly, over weeks to several months, where bone will grow from one level, to the next, forming a solid bridge of bone. This is why physicians obtain x-rays (radiographs) after a fusion surgery to observe for possible indicators of fusion. In patients with osteoporosis, the process of bone growth is less vigorous, and a condition called pseudoarthrosis can occur, where bone

---

[17] Motion segment: two contiguous vertebra including the intervertebral disc. Eg. A fusion procedure of L4 and L5 is a one-level fusion, as this involves stabilization of one motion segment. The anterior portion of the spine has one disc space in a motion segment, whereas there are two facet joints (right and left) that separate adjacent segments in the posterior aspect of L4 and L5.

does not form a bridge across. Signs of a failure of fusion to occur may be persistent or worsening back pain, or even complications with the hardware, such as screw or rod breakage or migration.

Another consideration with compression fractures is the variability in surgeon decision-making. Any discussion of surgical indications would over trivialize several key matters in the attempt to keep this book concise and relevant for a wide audience, general spinal surgery books such as the two volume, *Benzel's Spine Surgery*, exceeding 1800 pages.

Do any of the above medications to treat osteoporosis result in an increase in fusion success if given around the time of surgery?

At the present time, there is insufficient evidence that any of these medications increase fusion success.

However, there may be some benefit with the use of teriparatide. In 1 study, teriparatide was administered to postmenopausal women with a low bone mineral density that underwent 1 or 2 level posterior lateral lumbar fusion. They were given teriparatide to months prior to surgery and an average of 8 weeks following surgery. The 2 groups of 5057 women received either 20 mcg/day and the other half received 17.5 mg/week of the oral bisphosphonate medication risedronate. One year follow-up the rate of fusion was 82% versus 68% in the teriparatide versus risedronate groups, respectively. This suggests a benefit of teriparatide over bisphosphonate. However, the study did not compare fusion rates between medications that increase bone mineral density and placebo.[263]

Another study evaluated pedicle screw loosening in postmenopausal women that were treated out with either teriparatide, risedronate, and a control group that did not receive any treatment. At 1 year, by CT, the radial screw loosening was 13% and the teriparatide group and 26% in the bisphosphonate group as well as 25% in the placebo group. This suggests that teriparatide is slightly more effective at preventing screw loosening however this study suffers from a weak design due to a small patient population. Small differences in these patient populations can confound the results. However, these results are promising.[264]

Other issues when considering these studies and the benefits of spinal surgery comes from ensuring that that the spinal surgery of interest is consistent. Many studies focus on long segment fusions which have higher non-union rates. These the surgeries that surgeons are always looking for ways to improve successful outcomes, especially the fusion rates. Therefore, when reading that vitamin D3 preoperative blood labs may improve fusion in scoliosis correction surgery, perhaps the treatment effect will be minimal for a one-level fusion surgery? Ultimately, understanding the issues of surgery is a herculean task and will require the effort of family, friends, and trusted healthcare providers.

15 Conclusions

As one can see, the management of osteoporosis is both complex and lacking in any consensus. The number of studies in this book may seem overwhelming, so some basic summary recommendations will be provided here. Unfortunately, there are very few generalizations when it comes to optimal workup, diagnosis, and treatment, and the best care is always an individualized treatment that takes into consideration all ones unique patient-specific history and problems. Osteoporosis is an epidemic in North America, and unfortunately, it is truly a disease that requires preventative treatment, but receives very little attention.

Just reading this book is a huge step towards making informed decisions. Due to the level of detail in the book, the following few pages will summarize some very important points regarding the risk factors, diagnosis, and treatment of osteoporosis.

Risk Factors

Identifying non-modifiable risk factor are important so that even patients who see themselves as healthy, could still be at risk for osteoporosis. Women, especially post-menopausal women are at a greater risk than men. Generally, Caucasians, Asians, those with a family history of osteoporosis, and a low body weight are likewise at risk. Eventually, with time, Men and particularly those with low testosterone are a greater risk for osteoporosis.

Lifestyle measures such as smoking, chronic alcohol abuse, nutrient poor diets (junk food, inadequate or excessive calories, low calcium and vitamin D), as well as a general sedentary lifestyle, devoid of general outdoor or physical activity, constitute risks for osteoporosis and thus needs to be addressed— also for a myriad of other health reasons.

Certain medications for major medical problems will need an individualized approach to monitor for or treat osteoporosis. These include treatment for hypothyroidism, chronic steroid use, heparin use, and certain seizure medication can all potentially lower bone mineral density.

Formal Diagnosis

Despite the shortcomings of bone densitometry, diagnosis is based off of a T-score 'Normal' being +2.5 to -1 (SD), -1 to -2.5 being osteopenia, and less than -2.5 SD being a diagnosis of osteoporosis. This is a widely observed World Health Organization recommendation although "bone quality" research finds spinal lumbar T-scores to have a high variability and not correlate well with spinal fracture risk. Despite this, it is predictive of hip fracture risk, which carries a high mortality.

Medical Management

Most adults are deficient in calcium and vitamin D to an overreliance on cheap, nutrient-poor processed foods. Daily calcium intake for adults is recommended by the NIH to be at the minimum of one gram of calcium and 4,000 IU daily.

Non-Pharmacologic

Avoiding osteoporosis requires healthy living, and an observance of the risk factors stated above. While exercise and weight loss have conflicting evidence in the literature, there is an abundance of research that supports exercise and maintaining a healthy weight. Excess exercise and dieting places burdens on metabolic needs and appears to favor the breakdown of bone as well as promotes bone turnover at a rate that may exceed one's daily nutrition.

Pharmacologic

There are numerous FDA-approved osteoporosis medications that have strengths and weaknesses. In general, medications vary in terms of their efficacy, measured as their relative bone-building ability. The more imminent one's fracture risk, such as a T-score less than -3, or a recent diagnosis of a spinal compression fracture and T-score less than -2.5, the stronger the class of medication one will be prescribed. A number of variables make it impossible to predict accurately what the best medication may be for someone with osteoporosis due to the numerous primary and secondary causes of osteoporosis, and other medical problems that may make someone a high risk for adverse effects of a certain medication. Some very specific, and severe potential adverse risks are reported for many of these medications and in general the more effective the medication, the more potential for adverse effect. It is important to have a thorough understanding of these risks before beginning any treatment.

Compression Fractures

Compression fractures are a shortening of the vertebral body in the spine, and often commonly occur between T10 and L2 in the thoracolumbar region. However, compression fractures occur at just about all other levels. Shortening of the front of the spine causes spinal deformity, and is a risk for nerve compression. As assessment by a physician is required to make a plan of care urgently. Red flag symptoms include, but are not limited to, severe unrelenting pain with any movement, pain travelling down the legs (radicular pain), neurologic symptoms such as weakness, numbness, and bowel, bladder, or sexual dysfunction, which are all emergencies.

Bracing practices are highly variable and is often prescribed for compression fractures, with the goal to help with pain, and potentially avoid the development of worsening kyphosis. In a small fraction of patients with unrelenting pain despite medical management with medications and bracing, a vertebroplasty or kyphoplasty may be of benefit for some patients. Not all patients are a candidate due to specific anatomical concerns.

Lastly, despite this attempt to summarize the entire book in three pages, healthcare is incredibly complex and will invariably require the care of a trusted physician or health care provider whom the patient has developed a relationship with, and expects their care to be tailored to their goals and values.

16 Appendix

I. Cellular Phone Use, Electromagnetic Radiation, and Study of Effects on Bone Health

Cellular phones rely on radiofrequency radiation (RFR) to transmit information, along with a growing number of technologies that also rely on RFR. The National Environmental Policy Act of 1969 was created to monitor for potential impacts of the diversity of RFR and electromagnetic radiation that is in use today. So far, the official position of the CDC is that there are no identified adverse effects of RFR from cellular phones. In 2017, in asking the question, "Do cell phones pose a health hazard?", the CDC states,

> "At this time, **we do not have the science to link** health problems to cell phone use. Scientific studies are underway to determine whether cell phone use may cause health effects. It is also important to consider the benefits of cell phones. Their use can be valuable in an urgent or emergency situation – and even save lives."[265] (emphasis added)

There are numerous obstacles to proving the link between cell phone RFR and worsening bone health. First, 85% of American adults surveyed in 2021 state that they use a smart phone, according to one poll.[266] Determining cause-and-effect at the very least requires a control population , which would be people without cell phone use. The next hurdle is navigating the unknown dose-response relationship. The body contains numerous mechanisms for mitigating the effects of the many toxic compounds that we are exposed to. Ultimately, many compounds exist in such minute quantities that their negative effects are often not noticed. Cell phone usage varies, so the amount of radiofrequency radiation that is emitted from cellular phones varies per person. Also, the frequency and power, and the location on the body that a person wears a phone, or does not wear a phone varies significantly. Perhaps some cell phone cases or clothing can influence that exposure. The longer one thinks about the many variables involved, it becomes fairly understandable why proving this link is difficult. In answering the question, "Can using a cell phone cause cancer?", the CDC states, without using definitive terms (as in *yes* or *no*),

> "There is no scientific evidence that provides a definite answer to that question. Some organizations recommend caution in cell phone use. More research is needed before we know if using cell phones causes health effects."[267]

Other considerations

With that said, one study published in the *Journal of Craniofacial Surgery* suggested a potential association between cell phone pocket storage and decrease bone mineral density in the hip. However, comparing participants who worse cell phones in their pockets from 12 to 20 hours a day for a mean duration of 6 years did not show statistically significant difference in the bone density of those who consistently kept their cell phone at the level of the hip in belt holder or their pocket.[268] Overall, this study suffers many limitations in design, is limited in the number of participants, short duration, and lack of statistically significant findings. This means that the results may have arisen by chance alone, and not due to the studied exposure of cell phone radiation. Also, there is very little one can do in a study like this to account for other variables that impact one from developing osteoporosis. However, this association will certainly lead to further worry and investigation.

Conclusion: Insufficient Evidence Correlating EMR to Decreased Bone Health at This Time

At the present time, a definitive cause and effect relationship between EMR and worsened bone health. Serious challenges exist to measuring this exposure, let alone a cause-and-effect relationship between cell phone use and decreased bone mineral density or any other form of electromagnetic radiation. Were a relationship clearly shown in the future, it most likely would be a very weak relationship and thus a longer duration of study and larger population study would be two requirements to validate this hypothesis.

17 References

1 Wick, J. Y. Spontaneous fracture: multiple causes. *Consult Pharm* **24**, 100-102, 105-108, 110-102, doi:10.4140/tcp.n.2009.100 (2009).

2 Hatgis, J., Granville, M., Jacobson, R. E. & Berti, A. Sacral Insufficiency Fractures: Recognition and Treatment in Patients with Concurrent Lumbar Vertebral Compression Fractures. *Cureus* **9**, e1008, doi:10.7759/cureus.1008 (2017).

3 Erdem, Y. a. N., Cagri. Sneezing: A Rare Cause of Sacral Insufficiency Fracture in a Young Osteoporotic Woman. *Journal of Medical Cases* **5**, 159-162 (2017).

4 Jorgensen, N. R. *et al.* The prevalence of osteoporosis in patients with chronic obstructive pulmonary disease: a cross sectional study. *Respir Med* **101**, 177-185, doi:10.1016/j.rmed.2006.03.029 (2007).

5 *UAB Fragility Fracture Program Treats, Prevents Injuries Due to Weak Bones*

<https://www.uabmedicine.org/-/uab-fragility-fracture-program-treats-prevents-injuries-due-to-weak-bones> (2021).

6 Stone, A. A. & Broderick, J. E. Obesity and pain are associated in the United States. *Obesity (Silver Spring)* **20**, 1491-1495, doi:10.1038/oby.2011.397 (2012).

7 Frost, H. M. Bone's mechanostat: a 2003 update. *Anat Rec A Discov Mol Cell Evol Biol* **275**, 1081-1101, doi:10.1002/ar.a.10119 (2003).

8 Eimori, K. *et al.* Disrupted Bone Metabolism in Long-Term Bedridden Patients. *PLoS One* **11**, e0156991, doi:10.1371/journal.pone.0156991 (2016).

9 Administrator, N. C. *Preventing Bone Loss in Space Flight with Prophylactic Use of Bisphosphonate: Health Promotion of the Elderly by Space Medicine Technologies*, <https://www.nasa.gov/mission_pages/station/research/benefits/bone_loss.html> (2012).

10 Kelly, S. *Endurance: A year in space, a lifetime of discovery.* 174 (Knopf, 2017).

11 Walters, P. H., Jezequel, J. J. & Grove, M. B. Case study: Bone mineral density of two elite senior female powerlifters. *J Strength Cond Res* **26**, 867-872, doi:10.1519/JSC.0b013e31822c71c0 (2012).

12 Tsuzuku, S., Ikegami, Y. & Yabe, K. Effects of high-intensity resistance training on bone mineral density in young male powerlifters. *Calcif Tissue Int* **63**, 283-286, doi:10.1007/s002239900527 (1998).

13 Whyte, M. P. Misinterpretation of osteodensitometry with high bone density: BMD Z > or = + 2.5 is not "normal". *J Clin Densitom* **8**, 1-6, doi:10.1385/jcd:8:1:001 (2005).

14 Gregson, C. L., Hardcastle, S. A., Cooper, C. & Tobias, J. H. Friend or foe: high bone mineral density on routine bone density scanning, a review of causes and management. *Rheumatology (Oxford)* **52**, 968-985, doi:10.1093/rheumatology/ket007 (2013).

15 Briggs, A. M., Greig, A. M. & Wark, J. D. The vertebral fracture cascade in osteoporosis: a review of aetiopathogenesis. *Osteoporos Int* **18**, 575-584, doi:10.1007/s00198-006-0304-x (2007).

16 Christensen, D. L. *et al.* Proximal Femur Hounsfield Units on CT Colonoscopy Correlate With Dual-energy X-ray Absorptiometry. *Clin Orthop Relat Res* **477**, 850-860, doi:10.1097/CORR.0000000000000480 (2019).

17 Team, D. E. *These 5 Buildings Rocked Earthquake-Proof Designs*, <https://blog.dormakaba.com/these-5-buildings-rocked-earthquake-proof-designs/> (2019).

18 CDC. *Health Effects of Cigarette Smoking*, <https://www.cdc.gov/tobacco/data_statistics/fact_sheets/health_effects/effects_cig_smoking/index.htm> (2020).

19 HHS. *Informed Consent: Frequently Asked Questions*, <https://www.hhs.gov/ohrp/regulations-and-policy/guidance/faq/informed-consent/index.html> (2021).

20 Nijhawan, L. P. *et al.* Informed consent: Issues and challenges. *J Adv Pharm Technol Res* **4**, 134-140, doi:10.4103/2231-4040.116779 (2013).

21 Institute, L. I. 45 CFR § 46.116 - General requirements for informed consent. (2021).

22 Legg, T. J. *What You Need To Know About Informed Consent*, <https://www.healthline.com/health/informed-consent> (2019).

23 Merrill, R. K. *et al.* Negative Sagittal Balance Following Adult Spinal Deformity Surgery. *Global Spine J* **8**, 149-155, doi:10.1177/2192568217699187 (2018).

24 Kachlik, D., Varga, I., Baca, V. & Musil, V. Variant Anatomy and Its Terminology. *Medicina (Kaunas)* **56**, doi:10.3390/medicina56120713 (2020).

25 Bergman, J. *Useless Organs: The Rise and Fall of a Central Claim of Evolution* (BP Books, 2019).

26 Pillai, M. K. & Nair, S. T. A True Human Tail in a Neonate: Case report and literature review. *Sultan Qaboos Univ Med J* **17**, e109-e111, doi:10.18295/squmj.2016.17.01.020 (2017).

27 Woon, J. T., Perumal, V., Maigne, J. Y. & Stringer, M. D. CT morphology and morphometry of the normal adult coccyx. *Eur Spine J* **22**, 863-870, doi:10.1007/s00586-012-2595-2 (2013).

28 Apazidis, A., Ricart, P. A., Diefenbach, C. M. & Spivak, J. M. The prevalence of transitional vertebrae in the lumbar spine. *Spine J* **11**, 858-862, doi:10.1016/j.spinee.2011.08.005 (2011).

29 Mahato, N. K. Morphological traits in sacra associated with complete and partial lumbarization of first sacral segment. *Spine J* **10**, 910-915, doi:10.1016/j.spinee.2010.07.392 (2010).

30 Tang, M. *et al.* Lumbosacral transitional vertebra in a population-based study of 5860 individuals: prevalence and relationship to low back pain. *Eur J Radiol* **83**, 1679-1682, doi:10.1016/j.ejrad.2014.05.036 (2014).

31 Apaydin, M., Uluc, M. E. & Sezgin, G. Lumbosacral transitional vertebra in the young men population with low back pain: anatomical considerations and degenerations (transitional vertebra types in the young men population with low back pain). *Radiol Med* **124**, 375-381, doi:10.1007/s11547-018-0974-4 (2019).

32 Klibanski A et al. [NIH Consensus Development Panel on Osteoporosis Prevention, D., and Therapy]. Osteoporosis prevention, diagnosis, and therapy. *JAMA* **285**, 785-795 (2001).

33 Florencio-Silva R., e. a. Biology of Bone Tissue: Structure, Function, and Factors That Influence Bone Cells. *BioMed Research International* (2015).

34 Eriksen, E. F. Cellular mechanisms of bone remodeling. *Rev Endocr Metab Disord* **11**, 219-227, doi:10.1007/s11154-010-9153-1 (2010).

35 Wikipedia. *Robert Wadlow*, <https://en.wikipedia.org/wiki/Robert_Wadlow> (

36 Kacker, R., Conners, W., Zade, J. & Morgentaler, A. Bone mineral density and response to treatment in men younger than 50 years with testosterone deficiency and sexual dysfunction or infertility. *J Urol* **191**, 1072-1076, doi:10.1016/j.juro.2013.10.070 (2014).

37 Olney, R. C. Regulation of bone mass by growth hormone. *Med Pediatr Oncol* **41**, 228-234, doi:10.1002/mpo.10342 (2003).

38 Sheng, S.-R. Anatomy of large animal spines and its comparison to the human spine: a systematic review. *European Spine Journal* **19**, 46-56 (2010).

39 al., M. R. e. Comparative morphometry of L4 vertebrae: comparison of large animal models for the human lumbar spine. *Spine* **27**, E200-206 (2002).

40 Osterhoff, G. *et al.* Bone mechanical properties and changes with osteoporosis. *Injury* **47 Suppl 2**, S11-20, doi:10.1016/S0020-1383(16)47003-8 (2016).

41 Mittra, E., Rubin, C., Gruber, B. & Qin, Y. X. Evaluation of trabecular mechanical and microstructural properties in human calcaneal bone of advanced age using mechanical testing, microCT, and DXA. *J Biomech* **41**, 368-375, doi:10.1016/j.jbiomech.2007.09.003 (2008).

42 Burge, R. & al., e. Incidence and economic burden of osteoporosis-related fractures in the United States, 2005-2025. **22**, 465-475 (2007).

43 McCarthy, J. & Davis, A. Diagnosis and Management of Vertebral Compression Fractures. *Am Fam Physician* **94**, 44-50 (2016).

44 Dempster, D. W. in *AJMC* (2011).

45 Curry, S. Screening for osteoporosis to prevent fractures: US Preventative Services Task Force Recommendation Statement. **319**, 2521-2531 (2018).

46 in *International Osteoporosis Foundation.*

47 General, O. o. t. U. S. in *Bone Health and Osteoporosis: A Report of the Surgeon General Reports of the Surgeon General* (2004).

48 Schnell, S., Friedman, S. M., Mendelson, D. A., Bingham, K. W. & Kates, S. L. The 1-year mortality of patients treated in a hip fracture program for elders. *Geriatr Orthop Surg Rehabil* **1**, 6-14, doi:10.1177/2151458510378105 (2010).

49 Campbell, P. G. *et al.* Comparison of ICD-9-based, retrospective, and prospective assessments of perioperative complications: assessment of accuracy in reporting. *J Neurosurg Spine* **14**, 16-22, doi:10.3171/2010.9.SPINE10151 (2011).

50 *The Framingham Osteoporosis Study*, <https://www.ncbi.nlm.nih.gov/projects/gap/cgi-bin/study.cgi?study_id=phs000078.v2.p1> (

51 al., H. M. T. e. Risk Factors for Longitudinal Bone Loss in Elderly Men and Women: The Framingham Osteoporosis Study. *Journal of Bone and Mineral Research* **15**, 710-720 (2000).

52 CDC. *Smoking and Tobacco Use: Data and Statistics*, <https://www.cdc.gov/tobacco/data_statistics/index.htm> (2021).

53 Broulik, P. D., Rosenkrancova, J., Ruzicka, P., Sedlacek, R. & Kurcova, I. The effect of chronic nicotine administration on bone mineral content and bone strength in normal and castrated male rats. *Horm Metab Res* **39**, 20-24, doi:10.1055/s-2007-957342 (2007).

54 Huegel, J. *et al.* Chronic Nicotine Exposure Minimally Affects Rat Supraspinatus Tendon Properties and Bone Microstructure. *Ann Biomed Eng* **49**, 1333-1341, doi:10.1007/s10439-020-02667-x (2021).

55 Mito, K. *et al.* The nicotinic acetylcholine receptor alpha7 subunit is an essential negative regulator of bone mass. *Sci Rep* **7**, 45597, doi:10.1038/srep45597 (2017).

56 Jorde, R. *et al.* Smoking and other determinants of bone turnover. *PLoS One* **14**, e0225539, doi:10.1371/journal.pone.0225539 (2019).

57 Pennisi, E. Genomics. ENCODE project writes eulogy for junk DNA. *Science* **337**, 1159, 1161, doi:10.1126/science.337.6099.1159 (2012).

58 CDC. *Current Cigarette Smoking Among Adults in the United States*, <https://www.cdc.gov/tobacco/data_statistics/fact_sheets/adult_data/cig_smoking/index.htm> (2020).

59 Jensen, R. P., Luo, W., Pankow, J. F., Strongin, R. M. & Peyton, D. H. Hidden formaldehyde in e-cigarette

aerosols. *N Engl J Med* **372**, 392-394, doi:10.1056/NEJMc1413069 (2015).

60 Gennimata SA; Palamidas A; Kaltsakas G, e. a. Acute effect of e-cigarette on pulmonary function in healthy subjects and smokers. *European Respiratory Journal* **40** (2012).

61 Ambrose, B. K. *et al.* Flavored Tobacco Product Use Among US Youth Aged 12-17 Years, 2013-2014. *JAMA* **314**, 1871-1873, doi:10.1001/jama.2015.13802 (2015).

62 CDC. *E-cigarettes shaped like flash drives*, <https://www.cdc.gov/tobacco/infographics/youth/pdfs/e-cigarettes-usb-flash-508.pdf> (2020).

63 Langmaid, V. *E-cigarette company Juul to pay $40 million in North Carolina lawsuit settlement*, <https://www.cnn.com/2021/06/28/health/juul-north-carolina-lawsuit-settlement/index.html> (2021).

64 Reumann, M. K. *et al.* E-vapor aerosols do not compromise bone integrity relative to cigarette smoke after 6-month inhalation in an ApoE(-/-) mouse model. *Arch Toxicol* **94**, 2163-2177, doi:10.1007/s00204-020-02769-4 (2020).

65 Fiani, B. *et al.* The Impact of "Vaping" Electronic Cigarettes on Spine Health. *Cureus* **12**, e8907, doi:10.7759/cureus.8907 (2020).

66 CDC. Micronutrient Vitamins and Minerals. (2021).

67 Anderson, J. J., Roggenkamp, K. J. & Suchindran, C. M. Calcium intakes and femoral and lumbar bone density of elderly U.S. men and women: National Health and Nutrition Examination Survey 2005-2006 analysis. *J Clin Endocrinol Metab* **97**, 4531-4539, doi:10.1210/jc.2012-1407 (2012).

68 Tietz, T. *Elmer McCollum and the Discovery of Vitamins*, <http://scihi.org/elmer-collum-vitamins/> (2016).

69 Martins e Silva, J. [Brief history of rickets and of the discovery of vitamin D]. *Acta Reumatol Port* **32**, 205-229 (2007).

70 Moon, J. Y. a. R., C.J. *The Vitamin D-Problem An Important Lesson in Orthomolecular Medicine* <http://orthomolecular.org/library/jom/1975/pdf/1975-v04n02-p123.pdf> (1975).

71 Holick, M. F. Photosynthesis of vitamin D in the skin: effect of environmental and life-style variables. *Fed Proc* **46**, 1876-1882 (1987).

72 Sahni, S., Mangano, K. M., Kiel, D. P., Tucker, K. L. & Hannan, M. T. Dairy Intake Is Protective against Bone Loss in Older Vitamin D Supplement Users: The Framingham Study. *J Nutr* **147**, 645-652, doi:10.3945/jn.116.240390 (2017).

73 Mangano, K. M., Noel, S. E., Sahni, S. & Tucker, K. L. Higher Dairy Intakes Are Associated with Higher Bone Mineral Density among Adults with Sufficient Vitamin D Status: Results from the Boston Puerto Rican Osteoporosis Study. *J Nutr* **149**, 139-148, doi:10.1093/jn/nxy234 (2019).

74 Banerjee, T. *et al.* Dietary acid load and chronic kidney disease among adults in the United States. *BMC Nephrol* **15**, 137, doi:10.1186/1471-2369-15-137 (2014).

75 Hamm, L. L., Nakhoul, N. & Hering-Smith, K. S. Acid-Base Homeostasis. *Clin J Am Soc Nephrol* **10**, 2232-2242, doi:10.2215/CJN.07400715 (2015).

76 Qing, G. Z., Lu, Y., Yi, T., Zhang, K. Q. & Tang, Z. H. The relationship of frequency of meat consumption and osteoporosis in Chinese postmenopausal women. *Int J Clin Exp Med* **8**, 21130-21137 (2015).

77 Li, X., Lei, T., Tang, Z. & Dong, J. Analyzing the association between fish consumption and osteoporosis in a sample of Chinese men. *J Health Popul Nutr* **36**, 13, doi:10.1186/s41043-017-0088-y (2017).

78 Ho, S. C. *et al.* Soy protein consumption and bone mass in early postmenopausal Chinese women.

Osteoporos Int **14**, 835-842, doi:10.1007/s00198-003-1453-9 (2003).

79 Liu, N., Zeng, F., Zhang, K. & Tang, Z. A community-based cross-sectional study for relationship of frequency of vegetables intake and osteoporosis in a Chinese postmenopausal women sample. *BMC Womens Health* **16**, 28, doi:10.1186/s12905-016-0307-5 (2016).

80 van den Heuvel, E. & Steijns, J. Dairy products and bone health: how strong is the scientific evidence? *Nutr Res Rev* **31**, 164-178, doi:10.1017/S095442241800001X (2018).

81 Sahni, S. *et al.* Protective association of milk intake on the risk of hip fracture: results from the Framingham Original Cohort. *J Bone Miner Res* **29**, 1756-1762, doi:10.1002/jbmr.2219 (2014).

82 Tavani, A., Negri, E. & La Vecchia, C. Calcium, dairy products, and the risk of hip fracture in women in northern Italy. *Epidemiology* **6**, 554-557, doi:10.1097/00001648-199509000-00017 (1995).

83 McCabe, L. D. *et al.* Dairy intakes affect bone density in the elderly. *Am J Clin Nutr* **80**, 1066-1074, doi:10.1093/ajcn/80.4.1066 (2004).

84 Bian, S. *et al.* Dairy product consumption and risk of hip fracture: a systematic review and meta-analysis. *BMC Public Health* **18**, 165, doi:10.1186/s12889-018-5041-5 (2018).

85 *Fermentation*, <https://www.britannica.com/science/fermentation> (Adams, A; et al).

86 Parvaneh, K., Jamaluddin, R., Karimi, G. & Erfani, R. Effect of probiotics supplementation on bone mineral content and bone mass density. *ScientificWorldJournal* **2014**, 595962, doi:10.1155/2014/595962 (2014).

87 NIH. *Calcium and Vitamin D: Important and Every Age*, <https://www.bones.nih.gov/health-info/bone/bone-health/nutrition/calcium-and-vitamin-d-important-every-age> (2018).

88 Reddy, A. e. a. *The pH of Beverages In The United States*, <https://www.ada.org/en/~/media/ADA/Public%20Programs/Files/JADA_The%20pH%20of%20beverages%20in%20the%20United%20States> (2016).

89 University, C. *pH of Common Foods*, <https://www.clemson.edu/extension/food/food2market/documents/ph_of_common_foods.pdf> (

90 Juric A., e. a. *Analysis of total polyphenols, bitterness and haze in pale and dark lager beers produced under different mashing and boiling conditions*, <https://www.researchgate.net/figure/The-pH-colour-alcohol-and-CO-2-content-in-beers_tbl1_281897222> (

91 Butler, N. *Acidity in Tea: pH Levels, Effects, and More*, <https://www.healthline.com/health/food-nutrition/is-tea-acidic#ph-of-tea> (2017).

92 Ishimi, Y. Osteoporosis and Lifestyle. *J Nutr Sci Vitaminol (Tokyo)* **61 Suppl**, S139-141, doi:10.3177/jnsv.61.S139 (2015).

93 Tucker, K. L. *et al.* Colas, but not other carbonated beverages, are associated with low bone mineral density in older women: The Framingham Osteoporosis Study. *Am J Clin Nutr* **84**, 936-942, doi:10.1093/ajcn/84.4.936 (2006).

94 Dillman, D. A., Smith, Jolene, Melani, Leah. *Internet, phone, mail, and mixed-mode surveys: The tailored design method.* (Wiley Publishers, 2014).

95 Yoccuz, N. Use, Overuse, and Misuse of Significance Tests in Evolutionary Biology and Ec. *Bulletin of the Ecological Society of America* **72**, 106-111 (2010).

96 *24 Remarkable Caffeine Consumption Statistics*, <https://healthresearchfunding.org/remarkable-caffeine-consumption-statistics/> (2021).

97 Frary, C. D., Johnson, R. K. & Wang, M. Q. Food sources and intakes of caffeine in the diets of persons in the United States. *J Am Diet Assoc* **105**, 110-113, doi:10.1016/j.jada.2004.10.027 (2005).

98 *Spilling the Beans: How Much Caffeine is Too Much?*, <https://www.fda.gov/consumers/consumer-updates/spilling-beans-how-much-caffeine-too-much> (2018).

99 Choi, H., Choi, Y., Kim, J., Bae, J. & Roh, J. Longitudinal bone growth is impaired by direct involvement of caffeine with chondrocyte differentiation in the growth plate. *J Anat* **230**, 117-127, doi:10.1111/joa.12530 (2017).

100 Shin, J. *et al.* High doses of caffeine reduce in vivo osteogenic activity in prepubertal rats. *J Anat* **227**, 10-20, doi:10.1111/joa.12332 (2015).

101 Huang, T. H., Yang, R. S., Hsieh, S. S. & Liu, S. H. Effects of caffeine and exercise on the development of bone: a densitometric and histomorphometric study in young Wistar rats. *Bone* **30**, 293-299, doi:10.1016/s8756-3282(01)00659-7 (2002).

102 Forsmo, S., Schei, B., Langhammer, A. & Forsen, L. How do reproductive and lifestyle factors influence bone density in distal and ultradistal radius of early postmenopausal women? The Nord-Trondelag Health Survey, Norway. *Osteoporos Int* **12**, 222-229, doi:10.1007/s001980170133 (2001).

103 Rapuri, P. B., Gallagher, J. C. & Nawaz, Z. Caffeine decreases vitamin D receptor protein expression and 1,25(OH)2D3 stimulated alkaline phosphatase activity in human osteoblast cells. *J Steroid Biochem Mol Biol* **103**, 368-371, doi:10.1016/j.jsbmb.2006.12.037 (2007).

104 Yang, P., Zhang, X. Z., Zhang, K. & Tang, Z. Associations between frequency of coffee consumption and osteoporosis in Chinese postmenopausal women. *Int J Clin Exp Med* **8**, 15958-15966 (2015).

105 Corrao, G. *et al.* Coffee, caffeine, and the risk of liver cirrhosis. *Ann Epidemiol* **11**, 458-465, doi:10.1016/s1047-2797(01)00223-x (2001).

106 Chenoweth, M. J. *et al.* Analyses of nicotine metabolism biomarker genetics stratified by sex in

African and European Americans. *Sci Rep* **11**, 19572, doi:10.1038/s41598-021-98883-z (2021).

107 Chau, Y. P. *et al.* Serum Metabolome of Coffee Consumption and its Association With Bone Mineral Density: The Hong Kong Osteoporosis Study. *J Clin Endocrinol Metab* **105**, doi:10.1210/clinem/dgz210 (2020).

108 Choi, E. *et al.* The Benefit of Bone Health by Drinking Coffee among Korean Postmenopausal Women: A Cross-Sectional Analysis of the Fourth & Fifth Korea National Health and Nutrition Examination Surveys. *PLoS One* **11**, e0147762, doi:10.1371/journal.pone.0147762 (2016).

109 Tavani, A., Negri, E. & La Vecchia, C. Coffee intake and risk of hip fracture in women in northern Italy. *Prev Med* **24**, 396-400, doi:10.1006/pmed.1995.1064 (1995).

110 Li, X. L. & Xu, J. H. Coffee consumption and hip fracture risk: a meta-analysis. *J Nutr Sci* **2**, e23, doi:10.1017/jns.2013.13 (2013).

111 Yan, A., Zhang, H. H., Wang, S. Q. & Zhao, Y. Does tea consumption correlate to risk of fracture? A meta-analysis. *Int J Clin Exp Med* **8**, 8347-8357 (2015).

112 Xiang, W., Gu, K., Wang, W. & Jiang, X. Tea consumption and risk of fractures: an updated meta-analysis. *Osteoporos Int* **30**, 1941-1951, doi:10.1007/s00198-019-05095-3 (2019).

113 Tang, G. Y. *et al.* Phytochemical Composition and Antioxidant Capacity of 30 Chinese Teas. *Antioxidants (Basel)* **8**, doi:10.3390/antiox8060180 (2019).

114 Kuroyanagi, G. *et al.* (-)-Epigallocatechin gallate synergistically potentiates prostaglandin E2-stimulated osteoprotegerin synthesis in osteoblasts. *Prostaglandins Other Lipid Mediat* **128-129**, 27-33, doi:10.1016/j.prostaglandins.2017.02.001 (2017).

115 Huang, H. T. *et al.* Osteoprotective Roles of Green Tea Catechins. *Antioxidants (Basel)* **9**, doi:10.3390/antiox9111136 (2020).

116 *The 4 most important types of exercise* <https://www.health.harvard.edu/exercise-and-fitness/the-4-most-important-types-of-exercise> (2019).

117 Iwamoto, J. *et al.* Effects of treadmill exercise on bone mass, bone metabolism, and calciotropic hormones in young growing rats. *J Bone Miner Metab* **22**, 26-31, doi:10.1007/s00774-003-0443-5 (2004).

118 Kemmler, W., von Stengel, S., Engelke, K., Haberle, L. & Kalender, W. A. Exercise effects on bone mineral density, falls, coronary risk factors, and health care costs in older women: the randomized controlled senior fitness and prevention (SEFIP) study. *Arch Intern Med* **170**, 179-185, doi:10.1001/archinternmed.2009.499 (2010).

119 Korpelainen, R. *et al.* Long-term outcomes of exercise: follow-up of a randomized trial in older women with osteopenia. *Arch Intern Med* **170**, 1548-1556, doi:10.1001/archinternmed.2010.311 (2010).

120 Kemmler, W., Kohl, M. & von Stengel, S. Long-term effects of exercise in postmenopausal women: 16-year results of the Erlangen Fitness and Osteoporosis Prevention Study (EFOPS). *Menopause* **24**, 45-51, doi:10.1097/GME.0000000000000720 (2017).

121 O'Brien, M. Exercise and osteoporosis. *Ir J Med Sci* **170**, 58-62, doi:10.1007/BF03167724 (2001).

122 Berchtold, M. W., Brinkmeier, H. & Muntener, M. Calcium ion in skeletal muscle: its crucial role for muscle function, plasticity, and disease. *Physiol Rev* **80**, 1215-1265, doi:10.1152/physrev.2000.80.3.1215 (2000).

123 Voss, L. A., Fadale, P. D. & Hulstyn, M. J. Exercise-induced loss of bone density in athletes. *J Am Acad Orthop Surg* **6**, 349-357, doi:10.5435/00124635-199811000-00003 (1998).

124 De Souza, M. J. & Williams, N. I. Beyond hypoestrogenism in amenorrheic athletes: energy deficiency as a contributing factor for bone loss. *Curr Sports Med Rep* **4**, 38-44, doi:10.1007/s11932-005-0029-1 (2005).

125 Dawson-Hughes, B. *et al.* The potential impact of new National Osteoporosis Foundation guidance on treatment patterns. *Osteoporos Int* **21**, 41-52, doi:10.1007/s00198-009-1034-7 (2010).

126 U.S. Preventative Services Task Force: Screening For Osteoporosis To Prevent Fractures: Recommendation Statement. *American Family Physician* **98**, 594A (2018).

127 Force, U. S. P. S. T. *et al.* Screening for Osteoporosis to Prevent Fractures: US Preventive Services Task Force Recommendation Statement. *JAMA* **319**, 2521-2531, doi:10.1001/jama.2018.7498 (2018).

128 Eastell, R. *et al.* Pharmacological Management of Osteoporosis in Postmenopausal Women: An Endocrine Society* Clinical Practice Guideline. *J Clin Endocrinol Metab* **104**, 1595-1622, doi:10.1210/jc.2019-00221 (2019).

129 Camacho, P. M. *et al.* American Association of Clinical Endocrinologists and American College of Endocrinology Clinical Practice Guidelines for the Diagnosis and Treatment of Postmenopausal Osteoporosis - 2016. *Endocr Pract* **22**, 1-42, doi:10.4158/EP161435.GL (2016).

130 Buckley, L. *et al.* 2017 American College of Rheumatology Guideline for the Prevention and Treatment of Glucocorticoid-Induced Osteoporosis. *Arthritis Rheumatol* **69**, 1521-1537, doi:10.1002/art.40137 (2017).

131 Kanis, J. A., Cooper, C., Rizzoli, R. & Reginster, J. Y. Review of the guideline of the American College of Physicians on the treatment of osteoporosis. *Osteoporos Int* **29**, 1505-1510, doi:10.1007/s00198-018-4504-y (2018).

132 Kanis, J. A. *et al.* European guidance for the diagnosis and management of osteoporosis in postmenopausal women. *Osteoporos Int* **24**, 23-57, doi:10.1007/s00198-012-2074-y (2013).

133 Rossini, M. *et al.* Guidelines for the diagnosis, prevention and management of osteoporosis. *Reumatismo* **68**, 1-39, doi:10.4081/reumatismo.2016.870 (2016).

134 Center for Metabolic Bone Diseases, U. o. S., UK. *FRAX: Frequently Asked Questions*, <https://www.sheffield.ac.uk/FRAX/faq.aspx> (

135 Looker AC, e. a. FRAX-based Estimates of 10-year Probability of Hip and Major Osteoporotic Fracture Among Adults Aged 40 and Over: United States, 2013 and 2014 *National Health Statistics Report*, 6 (2017).

136 Ogden CL, C. M. *Prevalence of Overweight, Obesity, and Extreme Obesity Among Adults: United States, Trends 1960–1962 Through 2007–2008*, <https://www.cdc.gov/nchs/data/hestat/obesity_adult_07_08/obesity_adult_07_08.htm> (2010).

137 Looker AC, e. a. Osteoporosis or Low Bone Mass at the Femur Neck or Lumbar Spine in Older Adults: United States, 2005–2008. *NCHS Data Brief*, 1 (2012).

138 Lappe, J. M., Stegman, M. R. & Recker, R. R. The impact of lifestyle factors on stress fractures in female Army recruits. *Osteoporos Int* **12**, 35-42, doi:10.1007/s001980170155 (2001).

139 Lappe, J. *et al.* Calcium and vitamin d supplementation decreases incidence of stress fractures in female navy recruits. *J Bone Miner Res* **23**, 741-749, doi:10.1359/jbmr.080102 (2008).

140 Hertling, M. Obesity Is A National Security Issue - Presentation by Lt. Gen (Ret.) Mark Hertling.

141 M, K. J. a. B. *The Evolution of BMI values of US adults: 1882-1986*, <https://voxeu.org/article/100-years-us-obesity> (2010).

142 al, C. J. e. Obesity Is Not Protective against Fracture in Postmenopausal Women: GLOW. *The American Journal of Medicine* **124**, 1043-1050.

143 Bredella, M. A. *et al.* Determinants of bone microarchitecture and mechanical properties in obese men. *J Clin Endocrinol Metab* **97**, 4115-4122, doi:10.1210/jc.2012-2246 (2012).

144 Bredella, M. A. *et al.* Determinants of bone mineral density in obese premenopausal women. *Bone* **48**, 748-754, doi:10.1016/j.bone.2010.12.011 (2011).

145 Kajiki, Y. *et al.* Psoas muscle index predicts osteoporosis and fracture risk in individuals with degenerative spinal disease. *Nutrition* **93**, 111428, doi:10.1016/j.nut.2021.111428 (2021).

146 Korvala, J. *et al.* Genetic predisposition for femoral neck stress fractures in military conscripts. *BMC Genet* **11**, 95, doi:10.1186/1471-2156-11-95 (2010).

147 Mikkola, T. M. *et al.* Genetic and environmental influence on structural strength of weight-bearing and non-weight-bearing bone: a twin study. *J Bone Miner Res* **23**, 492-498, doi:10.1359/jbmr.071205 (2008).

148 Graham, S. *Identical Twins Exhibit Differences in Gene Expression*, <https://www.scientificamerican.com/article/identical-twins-exhibit-d/> (2005).

149 A, C. *Identical Twins are Not Identical*, <https://www.scientificamerican.com/article/identical-twins-genes-are-not-identical/> (2008).

150 Jonsson, H. *et al.* Differences between germline genomes of monozygotic twins. *Nat Genet* **53**, 27-34, doi:10.1038/s41588-020-00755-1 (2021).

151 *What is DNA?*, <https://medlineplus.gov/genetics/understanding/basics/dna/> (2021).

152 Nowak, R. *Mining Treasures from "Junk DNA"*, <https://www.science.org/doi/10.1126/science.7508142> (1994).

153 ME, D. *Junk DNA is not Junk*, <https://www.mdpi.com/journal/genes/special_issues/junk_DNA> (2012).

154 F, D. P. *What Junk DNA? It's an Operating System*, <https://www.genengnews.com/insights/what-junk-dna-its-an-operating-system/> (2013).

155 M, R. Guidelines for the diagnosis, prevention and management of osteoporosis. **68**, 1-39 (2016).

156 Mirza, F. & Canalis, E. Management of endocrine disease: Secondary osteoporosis: pathophysiology and management. *Eur J Endocrinol* **173**, R131-151, doi:10.1530/EJE-15-0118 (2015).

157 Nuti, R., Brandi, M., G, C. & al., e. Guidelines for the management of osteoporosis and fragility fractures. **14**, 86-88 (2019).

158 Berkheiser, K. in *Healthline* (2020).

159 in *NIH*.

160 Puttapitakpong, P. *et al.* Inter-correlation of knowledge, attitude, and osteoporosis preventive behaviors in women around the age of peak bone mass. *BMC Womens Health* **14**, 35, doi:10.1186/1472-6874-14-35 (2014).

161 Briot, K. DXA parameters: beyond bone mineral density. *Joint Bone Spine* **80**, 265-269, doi:10.1016/j.jbspin.2012.09.025 (2013).

162 Lewiecki, E. M. & Lane, N. E. Common mistakes in the clinical use of bone mineral density testing. *Nat Clin Pract Rheumatol* **4**, 667-674, doi:10.1038/ncprheum0928 (2008).

163 Lewiecki, E. M., Binkley, N. & Petak, S. M. DXA quality matters. *J Clin Densitom* **9**, 388-392, doi:10.1016/j.jocd.2006.07.002 (2006).

164 Pumberger, M. *et al.* Dual-energy X-ray Absorptiometry Does Not Represent Bone Structure in Patients with Osteoporosis: A Comparison of Lumbar Dual-Energy X-Ray Absorptiometry with Vertebral Biopsies. *Spine (Phila Pa 1976)* **46**, 861-866, doi:10.1097/BRS.0000000000003917 (2021).

165 Novo Matos, J. *et al.* Micro-computed tomography (micro-CT) for the assessment of myocardial disarray, fibrosis and ventricular mass in a feline model of hypertrophic cardiomyopathy. *Sci Rep* **10**, 20169, doi:10.1038/s41598-020-76809-5 (2020).

166 Pumberger, M. *et al.* Bone structure determined by HR-MDCT does not correlate with micro-CT of lumbar vertebral biopsies: a prospective cross-sectional human in vivo study. *J Orthop Surg Res* **15**, 398, doi:10.1186/s13018-020-01895-0 (2020).

167 USPSTF. *Clinician Summary of USPSTF Recommendation: Screening for Colorectal Cancer*, <file:///C:/Users/georg/AppData/Local/Temp/colorectal-cancer-screening-final-rec-clinician-summary.pdf> (2021).

168 Bolliger, S. e. a. Is Differentiation of Frequently Encountered Foreign Bodies in Corpses Possible by Hounsfield Density Measurement. *Journal of Forensic Sciences* **54**, 1119-1122 (2009).

169 Pinto, E. M. *et al.* Efficacy of Hounsfield Units Measured by Lumbar Computer Tomography on Bone Density Assessment: A Systematic Review. *Spine (Phila Pa 1976)*, doi:10.1097/BRS.0000000000004211 (2021).

170 Gucuk, A. & Uyeturk, U. Usefulness of hounsfield unit and density in the assessment and treatment of urinary stones. *World J Nephrol* **3**, 282-286, doi:10.5527/wjn.v3.i4.282 (2014).

171 Ahern, D. P. *et al.* A meta-analysis of the diagnostic accuracy of Hounsfield units on computed topography relative to dual-energy X-ray absorptiometry for the diagnosis of osteoporosis in the spine surgery population. *Spine J* **21**, 1738-1749, doi:10.1016/j.spinee.2021.03.008 (2021).

172 Graffy, P. M., Lee, S. J., Ziemlewicz, T. J. & Pickhardt, P. J. Prevalence of Vertebral Compression Fractures on Routine CT Scans According to L1 Trabecular Attenuation: Determining Relevant

Thresholds for Opportunistic Osteoporosis Screening. *AJR Am J Roentgenol* **209**, 491-496, doi:10.2214/AJR.17.17853 (2017).

173 Lee, S. J. *et al.* Opportunistic screening for osteoporosis using the sagittal reconstruction from routine abdominal CT for combined assessment of vertebral fractures and density. *Osteoporos Int* **27**, 1131-1136, doi:10.1007/s00198-015-3318-4 (2016).

174 Alacreu, E., Moratal, D. & Arana, E. Opportunistic screening for osteoporosis by routine CT in Southern Europe. *Osteoporos Int* **28**, 983-990, doi:10.1007/s00198-016-3804-3 (2017).

175 Marinova, M. *et al.* Use of routine thoracic and abdominal computed tomography scans for assessing bone mineral density and detecting osteoporosis. *Curr Med Res Opin* **31**, 1871-1881, doi:10.1185/03007995.2015.1074892 (2015).

176 St Jeor, J. D. *et al.* Average Lumbar Hounsfield Units Predicts Osteoporosis-Related Complications Following Lumbar Spine Fusion. *Global Spine J*, 2192568220975365, doi:10.1177/2192568220975365 (2020).

177 Lee, S. J., Anderson, P. A. & Pickhardt, P. J. Predicting Future Hip Fractures on Routine Abdominal CT Using Opportunistic Osteoporosis Screening Measures: A Matched Case-Control Study. *AJR Am J Roentgenol* **209**, 395-402, doi:10.2214/AJR.17.17820 (2017).

178 Bjerke, B. T. *et al.* Incidence of Osteoporosis-Related Complications Following Posterior Lumbar Fusion. *Global Spine J* **8**, 563-569, doi:10.1177/2192568217743727 (2018).

179 *Grading of Treatment Recommendations*, <https://www.uspreventiveservicestaskforce.org/uspstf/grade-definitions#july2012 > (2012).

180 United States preventive services task force: Screening for osteoporosis to prevent fractures: Recommendation statement. . *American Family Physician* **98**, 594A (2018).

181 Pickhardt, P. J. Opoortunistic Screening for Osteoporosis Using Abdominal Computed Tomography Scans Obtained for Other Indications. *Ann Intern Med* **158**, 588-595 (2013).

182 Nut, R. e. a. Guidelines for the management of osteoporosis and fragility fractures. *Internal and Emergency Medicine* **14**, 85-102 (2019).

183 Fardet, L., Petersen, I. & Nazareth, I. Monitoring of patients on long-term glucocorticoid therapy: a population-based cohort study. *Medicine (Baltimore)* **94**, e647, doi:10.1097/MD.0000000000000647 (2015).

184 Bazelier, M. T. *et al.* A simple score for estimating the long-term risk of fracture in patients with multiple sclerosis. *Neurology* **79**, 922-928, doi:10.1212/WNL.0b013e318266faae (2012).

185 De Vries, F. *et al.* Fracture risk with intermittent high-dose oral glucocorticoid therapy. *Arthritis Rheum* **56**, 208-214, doi:10.1002/art.22294 (2007).

186 Oshagbemi, O. A. *et al.* Use of high-dose intermittent systemic glucocorticoids and the risk of fracture in patients with chronic obstructive pulmonary disease. *Bone* **110**, 238-243, doi:10.1016/j.bone.2018.02.007 (2018).

187 van Staa, T. P. *et al.* A simple clinical score for estimating the long-term risk of fracture in post-menopausal women. *QJM* **99**, 673-682, doi:10.1093/qjmed/hcl094 (2006).

188 van Staa, T. P. *et al.* A simple score for estimating the long-term risk of fracture in patients using oral glucocorticoids. *QJM* **98**, 191-198, doi:10.1093/qjmed/hci029 (2005).

189 Laan, R. F. *et al.* Low-dose prednisone induces rapid reversible axial bone loss in patients with rheumatoid arthritis. A randomized, controlled study. *Ann Intern Med* **119**, 963-968, doi:10.7326/0003-4819-119-10-199311150-00001 (1993).

190 Canalis, E. Mechanisms of glucocorticoid-induced osteoporosis. *Curr Opin Rheumatol* **15**, 454-457, doi:10.1097/00002281-200307000-00013 (2003).

191 Kendler, D. e. a. Denosumab in the Treatment of Osteoporosis: 10 Years Later: A Narrative Review. *Advances in Therapy* (2021).

192 Girotra, M., Rubin, M. R. & Bilezikian, J. P. Anabolic Agents for Osteoporosis : What is Their Likely Place in Therapy? *Treat Endocrinol* **5**, 347-358, doi:10.2165/00024677-200605060-00003 (2006).

193 Reginster, J. Y. Strontium ranelate in osteoporosis. *Curr Pharm Des* **8**, 1907-1916, doi:10.2174/1381612023393639 (2002).

194 Sun, Y. *et al.* Strontium ranelate incorporated 3D porous sulfonated PEEK simulating MC3T3-E1 cell differentiation. *Regen Biomater* **8**, rbaa043, doi:10.1093/rb/rbaa043 (2021).

195 FitzGerald, P. *Why Strontium Is Not Advised for Bone Health*, <https://americanbonehealth.org/medications-bone-health/why-strontium-is-not-advised-for-bone-health/> (2020).

196 Eriksen, E. F. & Robins, D. A. Teriparatide: A bone formation treatment for osteoporosis. *Drugs Today (Barc)* **40**, 935-948, doi:10.1358/dot.2004.40.11.872582 (2004).

197 FDA. *FORTEO (TM) teriparatide (rDNA origin) injection 750 mcg/3mL* <https://www.accessdata.fda.gov/scripts/cder/daf/index.cfm?event=overview.process&ApplNo=021318> (2002).

198 Vahle, J. L. *et al.* Bone neoplasms in F344 rats given teriparatide [rhPTH(1-34)] are dependent on duration of treatment and dose. *Toxicol Pathol* **32**, 426-438, doi:10.1080/01926230490462138 (2004).

199 North American Menopause, S. Management of osteoporosis in postmenopausal women: 2006 position statement of The North American Menopause Society. *Menopause* **13**, 340-367; quiz

368-349, doi:10.1097/01.gme.0000222475.93345.b3 (2006).

200 Laura, I. *et al.* Which treatment to prevent an imminent fracture? *Bone Rep* **15**, 101105, doi:10.1016/j.bonr.2021.101105 (2021).

201 Chang, V. & Holly, L. T. Bracing for thoracolumbar fractures. *Neurosurg Focus* **37**, E3, doi:10.3171/2014.4.FOCUS1477 (2014).

202 Kweh, B. T. S. *et al.* The Role of Spinal Orthoses in Osteoporotic Vertebral Fractures of the Elderly Population (Age 60 Years or Older): Systematic Review. *Global Spine J* **11**, 975-987, doi:10.1177/2192568220948036 (2021).

203 Connolly, P. J. & Grob, D. Bracing of patients after fusion for degenerative problems of the lumbar spine--yes or no? *Spine (Phila Pa 1976)* **23**, 1426-1428, doi:10.1097/00007632-199806150-00024 (1998).

204 Hartshorne, E. On the causes and treatment of pseudarthrosis and especially that form of it sometimes called supernumerary joint. *Am J Med* **1**, 121-156 (1841).

205 *High-Frequency Pulsed Electromagnetic Stimulation* <https://www.aetna.com/cpb/medical/data/100_199/0175.html> (2021).

206 *National Coverage Determination: OSTEOGENIC STIMULATORs 150.2* <https://www.cms.gov/medicare-coverage-database/view/ncd.aspx?ncdid=65&ncdver=2&keyword=osteogenic%20stimulator&keywordType=starts&areaId=all&docType=NCA,CAL,NCD,MEDCAC,TA,MCD,6,3,5,1,F,P&contractOption=all&sortBy=relevance&bc=1> (2005).

207 Piazzolla, A. *et al.* Capacitive Coupling Electric Fields in the Treatment of Vertebral Compression Fractures. *J Biol Regul Homeost Agents* **29**, 637-646 (2015).

208 Kaiser, M. G. *et al.* Guideline update for the performance of fusion procedures for degenerative

disease of the lumbar spine. Part 17: bone growth stimulators as an adjunct for lumbar fusion. *J Neurosurg Spine* **21**, 133-139, doi:10.3171/2014.4.SPINE14326 (2014).

209 Mooney, V. A randomized double-blind prospective study of the efficacy of pulsed electromagnetic fields for interbody lumbar fusions. *Spine (Phila Pa 1976)* **15**, 708-712, doi:10.1097/00007632-199007000-00016 (1990).

210 Simmons, J. W., Jr., Mooney, V. & Thacker, I. Pseudarthrosis after lumbar spine fusion: nonoperative salvage with pulsed electromagnetic fields. *Am J Orthop (Belle Mead NJ)* **33**, 27-30 (2004).

211 Goldstein, C. L., Chutkan, N. B., Choma, T. J. & Orr, R. D. Management of the Elderly With Vertebral Compression Fractures. *Neurosurgery* **77 Suppl 4**, S33-45, doi:10.1227/NEU.0000000000000947 (2015).

212 Voormolen MH., e. a. Percutaneous vertebroplasty compared with optimal pain medication treatment: short-term clinical outcome of patients with subacute or chronic painful osteoporotic vertebral compression fractures- the VERTOS study. *AJNR Am J Neuroradiol* **28**, 555-560 (2007).

213 Ploeg WT, e. a. Percutaneeous vertebroplasty as a treatment for osteoporotic vertebral compression fractures: a systematic review. . *Eur Spine J* **15**, 1749-1758 (2006).

214 Klazen, C. A. *et al.* Clinical course of pain in acute osteoporotic vertebral compression fractures. *J Vasc Interv Radiol* **21**, 1405-1409, doi:10.1016/j.jvir.2010.05.018 (2010).

215 Venmans, A., Klazen, C. A., Lohle, P. N., Mali, W. P. & van Rooij, W. J. Natural history of pain in patients with conservatively treated osteoporotic vertebral compression fractures: results from VERTOS II. *AJNR Am J Neuroradiol* **33**, 519-521, doi:10.3174/ajnr.A2817 (2012).

216 Hayhurst, C. J. & Durieux, M. E. Differential Opioid Tolerance and Opioid-induced Hyperalgesia: A Clinical Reality. *Anesthesiology* **124**, 483-488, doi:10.1097/ALN.0000000000000963 (2016).

217 Guignard, B. *et al.* Acute opioid tolerance: intraoperative remifentanil increases postoperative pain and morphine requirement. *Anesthesiology* **93**, 409-417, doi:10.1097/00000542-200008000-00019 (2000).

218 Layton, K. F. *et al.* Vertebroplasty, first 1000 levels of a single center: evaluation of the outcomes and complications. *AJNR Am J Neuroradiol* **28**, 683-689 (2007).

219 Galibert P, e. a. Preliminary note on the treatment of vertebral angioma by percutaneous acrylic vertebroplasty [in French]. *Neurochirurgie* **33**, 166-168 (1987).

220 Predey, T. A., Sewall, L. E. & Smith, S. J. Percutaneous vertebroplasty: new treatment for vertebral compression fractures. *Am Fam Physician* **66**, 611-615 (2002).

221 Barzin, M. & Maleki, I. Incidence of vertebral hemangioma on spinal magnetic resonance imaging in Northern Iran. *Pak J Biol Sci* **12**, 542-544, doi:10.3923/pjbs.2009.542.544 (2009).

222 Piper, K. *et al.* Surgical Management and Adjuvant Therapy for Patients With Neurological Deficits From Vertebral Hemangiomas: A Meta-Analysis. *Spine (Phila Pa 1976)* **45**, E99-E110, doi:10.1097/BRS.0000000000003181 (2020).

223 Girardo, M. *et al.* Treatment of Aggressive Vertebral Hemangiomas with Poly Vinyl Alcohol (PVA) Microparticles Embolization, PMMA, and Short Segment Stabilization: Preliminary Results with at Least 5 Years of Follow-up. *World Neurosurg* **128**, e283-e288, doi:10.1016/j.wneu.2019.04.138 (2019).

224 Bafeta, A. *et al.* Impact of single centre status on estimates of intervention effects in trials with

continuous outcomes: meta-epidemiological study. *BMJ* **344**, e813, doi:10.1136/bmj.e813 (2012).

225 Bellomo, R., Warrillow, S. J. & Reade, M. C. Why we should be wary of single-center trials. *Crit Care Med* **37**, 3114-3119, doi:10.1097/CCM.0b013e3181bc7bd5 (2009).

226 Pocock, S. J. & Stone, G. W. The Primary Outcome Is Positive - Is That Good Enough? *N Engl J Med* **375**, 971-979, doi:10.1056/NEJMra1601511 (2016).

227 Lee, J. S., Hobden, E., Stiell, I. G. & Wells, G. A. Clinically important change in the visual analog scale after adequate pain control. *Acad Emerg Med* **10**, 1128-1130, doi:10.1111/j.1553-2712.2003.tb00586.x (2003).

228 Benhissen Z, e. a. Determining the minimal clinically important difference of the hand function sort questionnaire in vocational rehabilitation. *Annals of Physical and Rehabilitation Medicine* **62**, 155-160 (2019).

229 MacDowall, A., Skeppholm, M., Robinson, Y. & Olerud, C. Validation of the visual analog scale in the cervical spine. *J Neurosurg Spine* **28**, 227-235, doi:10.3171/2017.5.SPINE1732 (2018).

230 Association, A. P. *Criteria for Evaluating Treatment Guidelines*, <https://www.apa.org/practice/guidelines/evaluating> (2000).

231 Farrokhi, M. R., Alibai, E. & Maghami, Z. Randomized controlled trial of percutaneous vertebroplasty versus optimal medical management for the relief of pain and disability in acute osteoporotic vertebral compression fractures. *J Neurosurg Spine* **14**, 561-569, doi:10.3171/2010.12.SPINE10286 (2011).

232 Taylor, R. S., Taylor, R. J. & Fritzell, P. Balloon kyphoplasty and vertebroplasty for vertebral compression fractures: a comparative systematic review of efficacy and safety. *Spine (Phila Pa 1976)*

31, 2747-2755, doi:10.1097/01.brs.0000244639.71656.7d (2006).

233 Wang, H. *et al.* Comparison of Percutaneous Vertebroplasty and Balloon Kyphoplasty for the Treatment of Single Level Vertebral Compression Fractures: A Meta-analysis of the Literature. *Pain Physician* **18**, 209-222 (2015).

234 FDA. *Clinical Trial Considerations: Vertebral Augmentation Devices to Treat Spinal Insufficiency Fractures - Guidance for Industry and FDA Staff (Docket: FDA-2020-D-0957)*, <https://www.fda.gov/regulatory-information/search-fda-guidance-documents/clinical-trial-considerations-vertebral-augmentation-devices-treat-spinal-insufficiency-fractures#4G> (2004).

235 Al-Nakshabandi, N. A. Percutaneous vertebroplasty complications. *Ann Saudi Med* **31**, 294-297, doi:10.4103/0256-4947.81542 (2011).

236 Chen C., e. a. Intradural cement leakage after vertebroplasty. *The Spine Jouranl* **15**, 1493-1494 (2015).

237 Park, J. W. *et al.* Infection following percutaneous vertebral augmentation with polymethylmethacrylate. *Arch Osteoporos* **13**, 47, doi:10.1007/s11657-018-0468-y (2018).

238 Vasconcelos, C., Gailloud, P., Martin, J. B. & Murphy, K. J. Transient arterial hypotension induced by polymethylmethacrylate injection during percutaneous vertebroplasty. *J Vasc Interv Radiol* **12**, 1001-1002, doi:10.1016/s1051-0443(07)61584-x (2001).

239 Tozzi, P. *et al.* Management of pulmonary embolism during acrylic vertebroplasty. *Ann Thorac Surg* **74**, 1706-1708, doi:10.1016/s0003-4975(02)03962-0 (2002).

240 Ahmadzai, H., Campbell, S., Archis, C. & Clark, W. A. Fat embolism syndrome following percutaneous

vertebroplasty: a case report. *Spine J* **14**, e1-5, doi:10.1016/j.spinee.2013.09.021 (2014).

241 Kaufmann, T. J., Wald, J. T. & Kallmes, D. F. A technique to circumvent subcutaneous cement tracts during percutaneous vertebroplasty. *AJNR Am J Neuroradiol* **25**, 1595-1596 (2004).

242 Mooney, J., et al. Vertebral height restoration following kyphoplasty. *Journal of Spine Surgery* **5**, 194-200 (2019).

243 Lin, T. *et al.* Does spinal sagittal imbalance lead to future vertebral compression fractures in osteoporosis patients? *Spine J* **21**, 1362-1375, doi:10.1016/j.spinee.2021.03.014 (2021).

244 Schwab, F., Lafage, V., Boyce, R., Skalli, W. & Farcy, J. P. Gravity line analysis in adult volunteers: age-related correlation with spinal parameters, pelvic parameters, and foot position. *Spine (Phila Pa 1976)* **31**, E959-967, doi:10.1097/01.brs.0000248126.96737.0f (2006).

245 Wang, C. *et al.* Percutaneous kyphoplasty: Risk Factors for Recollapse of Cemented Vertebrae. *World Neurosurg* **130**, e307-e315, doi:10.1016/j.wneu.2019.06.071 (2019).

246 Heo, D. H., Chin, D. K., Yoon, Y. S. & Kuh, S. U. Recollapse of previous vertebral compression fracture after percutaneous vertebroplasty. *Osteoporos Int* **20**, 473-480, doi:10.1007/s00198-008-0682-3 (2009).

247 Yu, W., Xu, W., Jiang, X., Liang & Jian, W. Risk Factors for Recollapse of the Augmented Vertebrae After Percutaneous Vertebral Augmentation: A Systematic Review and Meta-Analysis. *World Neurosurg* **111**, 119-129, doi:10.1016/j.wneu.2017.12.019 (2018).

248 Niu, J. *et al.* Factors affecting recompression of augmented vertebrae after successful percutaneous balloon kyphoplasty: a retrospective analysis. *Acta Radiol* **56**, 1380-1387, doi:10.1177/0284185114556016 (2015).

249 Ha, K. Y. & Kim, Y. H. Risk factors affecting progressive collapse of acute osteoporotic spinal fractures. *Osteoporos Int* **24**, 1207-1213, doi:10.1007/s00198-012-2065-z (2013).

250 Wiggins, M. C., Sehizadeh, M., Pilgram, T. K. & Gilula, L. A. Importance of intravertebral fracture clefts in vertebroplasty outcome. *AJR Am J Roentgenol* **188**, 634-640, doi:10.2214/AJR.06.0542 (2007).

251 Lane, J. I. *et al.* Intravertebral clefts opacified during vertebroplasty: pathogenesis, technical implications, and prognostic significance. *AJNR Am J Neuroradiol* **23**, 1642-1646 (2002).

252 Vanni, D. *et al.* Third-generation percutaneous vertebral augmentation systems. *J Spine Surg* **2**, 13-20, doi:10.21037/jss.2016.02.01 (2016).

253 Werner, C. M. *et al.* Vertebral body stenting versus kyphoplasty for the treatment of osteoporotic vertebral compression fractures: a randomized trial. *J Bone Joint Surg Am* **95**, 577-584, doi:10.2106/JBJS.L.00024 (2013).

254 Singh, R. *et al.* Morphometric measurements of cadaveric thoracic spine in Indian population and its clinical applications. *Asian Spine J* **5**, 20-34, doi:10.4184/asj.2011.5.1.20 (2011).

255 Dublin, A. B., Hartman, J., Latchaw, R. E., Hald, J. K. & Reid, M. H. The vertebral body fracture in osteoporosis: restoration of height using percutaneous vertebroplasty. *AJNR Am J Neuroradiol* **26**, 489-492 (2005).

256 Teng, M. M. *et al.* Kyphosis correction and height restoration effects of percutaneous vertebroplasty. *AJNR Am J Neuroradiol* **24**, 1893-1900 (2003).

257 Chin, D. K., Kim, Y. S., Cho, Y. E. & Shin, J. J. Efficacy of postural reduction in osteoporotic vertebral compression fractures followed by percutaneous vertebroplasty. *Neurosurgery* **58**, 695-

700; discussion 695-700, doi:10.1227/01.NEU.0000204313.36531.79 (2006).

258 Hiwatashi, A., Moritani, T., Numaguchi, Y. & Westesson, P. L. Increase in vertebral body height after vertebroplasty. *AJNR Am J Neuroradiol* **24**, 185-189 (2003).

259 Muto, M. *et al.* Vertebral Body Stenting System for the Treatment of Osteoporotic Vertebral Compression Fracture: Follow-up at 12 Months in 20 Cases. *Neuroradiol J* **24**, 610-619, doi:10.1177/197140091102400418 (2011).

260 Ender, S. A. *et al.* Osseofix(R) system for percutaneous stabilization of osteoporotic and tumorous vertebral compression fractures - clinical and radiological results after 12 months. *Rofo* **186**, 380-387, doi:10.1055/s-0033-1355504 (2014).

261 Carman, D. L., Browne, R. H. & Birch, J. G. Measurement of scoliosis and kyphosis radiographs. Intraobserver and interobserver variation. *J Bone Joint Surg Am* **72**, 328-333 (1990).

262 Morrissy, R. T., Goldsmith, G. S., Hall, E. C., Kehl, D. & Cowie, G. H. Measurement of the Cobb angle on radiographs of patients who have scoliosis. Evaluation of intrinsic error. *J Bone Joint Surg Am* **72**, 320-327 (1990).

263 Polly, D. W., Jr. *et al.* Measurement of lumbar lordosis. Evaluation of intraobserver, interobserver, and technique variability. *Spine (Phila Pa 1976)* **21**, 1530-1535; discussion 1535-1536, doi:10.1097/00007632-199607010-00008 (1996).

264 Stotts, A. K., Smith, J. T., Santora, S. D., Roach, J. W. & D'Astous, J. L. Measurement of spinal kyphosis: implications for the management of Scheuermann's kyphosis. *Spine (Phila Pa 1976)* **27**, 2143-2146, doi:10.1097/00007632-200210010-00013 (2002).

265 Ohtori, S. *et al.* Teriparatide accelerates lumbar posterolateral fusion in women with postmenopausal osteoporosis: prospective study. *Spine (Phila Pa*

1976) **37**, E1464-1468, doi:10.1097/BRS.0b013e31826ca2a8 (2012).

266 Ohtori, S. *et al.* Comparison of teriparatide and bisphosphonate treatment to reduce pedicle screw loosening after lumbar spinal fusion surgery in postmenopausal women with osteoporosis from a bone quality perspective. *Spine (Phila Pa 1976)* **38**, E487-492, doi:10.1097/BRS.0b013e31828826dd (2013).

267 CDC. *Frequently Asked Questions About Cell phones and Your Health*, <https://www.cdc.gov/nceh/radiation/cell_phones._faq.html> (2017).

268 statista. *Percentage of U.S. adults who own a smartphone from 2011 to 2021*, <https://www.statista.com/statistics/219865/percentage-of-us-adults-who-own-a-smartphone/> (2021).

Index

Get These Other Fascinating Books by The Author on Amazon.com!

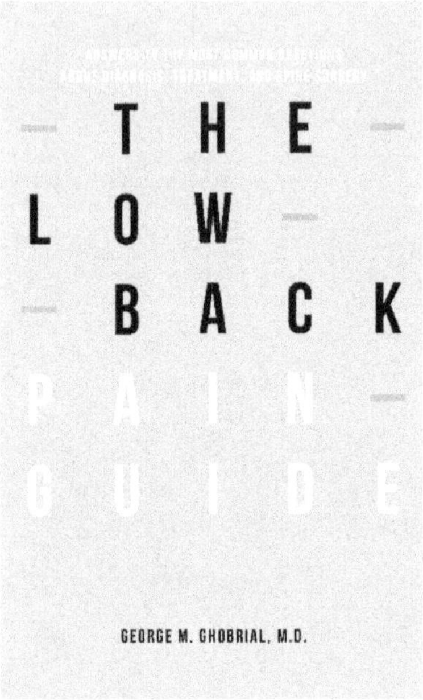

Suffering from low back pain and not sure where to get answers? Waking up in the morning with low back pain, or low back pain from sitting all day? The Low Back Pain Guide is your road map to getting well and your comprehensive reference book to diagnosing and managing low back pain, using a unique question and answer format. Answers To Over 50 Of the Most Common Questions !No Medical Background Required! Understand Causes of Back Pain, and Learn The Treatment Options With The Use of illustrations! Learn The Basics of Treating Modern Low Back Pain As Explained by A Neurosurgeon: Physical Therapy, Medication, Alternative Medicine, Injections, Basic Anatomy of the Spine,Diagnosis and Modern Imaging with X-ray, CT, MRI, Surgery, Stem Cells, and Laser Spine Surgery. IS LOW BACK PAIN TAKING OVER YOUR LIFE?Low back pain, or Lumbago, is among the most common medical problems facing us today, having the potential to affect every aspect of our lives. The process of obtaining pain relief is becoming increasingly complex. With The Low Back Pain Guide, take control of your healthcare and demystify the process of diagnosis and treatment. In this comprehensive and novel groundbreaking approach to patient medical education, the author outlines back pain treatment in a concise and illustrated Question and Answer Format. The author, a neurosurgeon, provides answers to more than 50 of the most frequently encountered questions, including relevant topics such as diagnostic imaging, physical therapy, medications, minimally-invasive surgery, laser spine surgery, spinal cord stimulation, and stem cell therapy. This is the most comprehensive guide to date. Take back control!

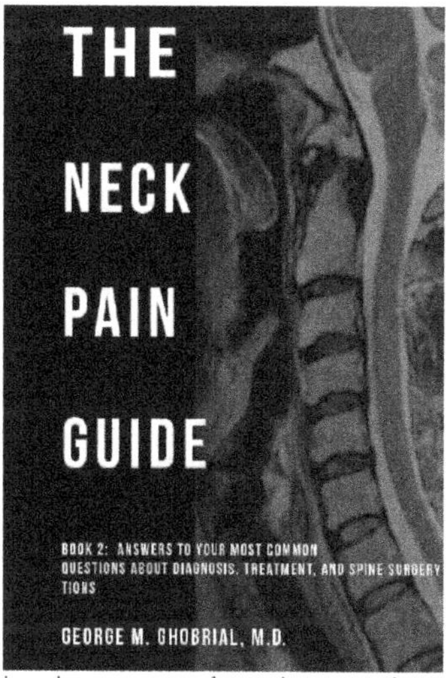

Dr. George M. Ghobrial's handbook for neck pain encompasses all aspects of diagnosis and care of acute and chronic neck pain: early and late management, resources, facilities, physicians and other healthcare providers and their roles, medication, physical therapy, imaging, as well as surgical and nonsurgical treatments. Using over 60 illustrations, Dr. Ghobrial introduces the anatomical and clinical issues related to degenerative disorders of the spine in a clear manner, explaining many terms such as disc herniations, spondylosis, degenerative disc disease, radiculopathy, and more. Topics include: common diagnostic imaging techniques such as X-ray, CT, MRI, as well as spinal injections, physical therapy, electrodiagnostic testing, discectomy, foraminotomy, laminotomy, fusion, disc replacement, scoliosis, bracing, minimally-invasive surgery, endoscopic surgery, laser spine surgery, and other emerging topics such as 'stem cell' injections and more. Suffering From Acute Neck and Arm Pain? Overwhelmed by the vast treatment options and not sure which to start with, or where to go? The Neck Pain Guide is a unique and comprehensive reference to assessing acute neck pain. Learn about concerning red flag symptoms, understand the available resources, and learn commonly avoidable options such as opiates and early imaging and invasive pain treatments. Having a medical background is not necessary to understand this book as the goal of this work is to educate patients and provide them with all the information in the same place, and to organize that information into a question and answer reference. Since not everyone has the precious free time to read lengthy nonfiction books on a single technical subject, this book is organized to allow for questions and topics to be more rapidly found among the table of contents and index, directing the reader to a helpful explanation and illustration. Despite being a highly prevalent healthcare problem in North America (also worldwide), there are no comprehensive, patient-centered books that cover the full scope of modern back pain management, which was the motivation for providing the Low Back Pain and Neck Pain Guides. Also, unlike the majority of patient-centered educational materials, a truly unique perspective is shared, which is that of a neurosurgeon with expertise and fellowship training in spinal surgery. This book will emphasize non-surgical treatments, since they comprise the majority of spinal care. The author, is a fellowship-trained spinal surgeon and neurosurgeon with an interest in public health and education. With that in mind, this book is for patients who wish to demystify neck and low back pain, critically assess their healthcare options, and maximize informed decision making.

Made in the USA
Monee, IL
04 November 2026

67378103R00125